THE QUICK AND EASY FOREVER STRONG DIET COOKBOOK

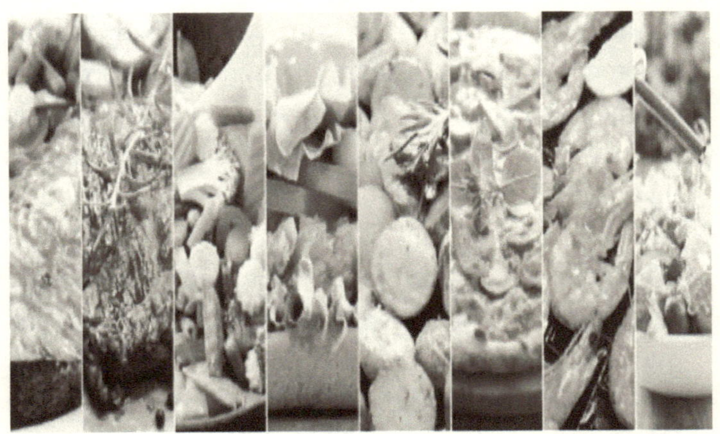

Discover The Brand New Tasty and Mouthwatering Science - Based Nutritious And Healthy Recipes That Will Make You Look Younger Forever

Kathleen Scribner

Copyright © [Kathleen Scribner], [2023]

Read more books by Kathleen Scribner by visiting:
https://www.amazon.com/author/skathleen234

TABLE OF CONTENTS

INTRODUCTION

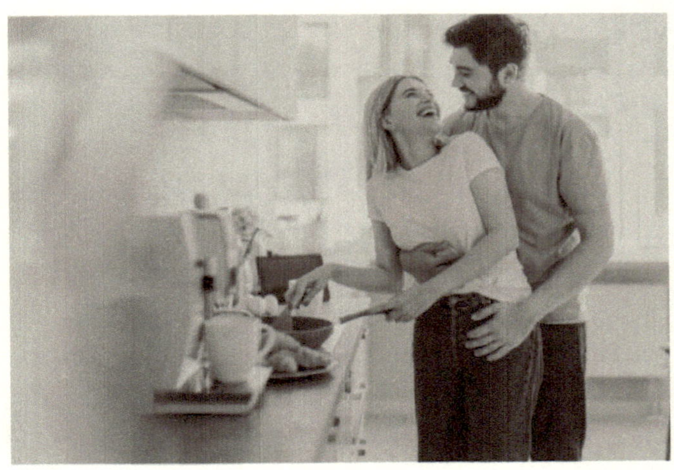

Welcome to "**The Quick And Easy Forever Strong Diet Cookbook:** *Discover The Brand New Tasty and Mouthwatering Science - Based Nutritious And Healthy Recipes That Will Make You Look Younger Forever."* In a world where the pursuit of eternal youth is a timeless aspiration, we are thrilled to embark on a culinary journey that not only tantalizes your taste buds but also promises to keep you looking and feeling youthful for years to come.

Aging is an inevitable part of life, but it doesn't have to be a relentless march toward diminished vitality and appearance. The food we consume plays a pivotal role in determining how we age. With the right nutrition, we have the power to slow down the clock, embrace our best selves, and age gracefully with confidence.

In this cookbook, we have curated a collection of delicious, nutritious, and scientifically-backed recipes designed to fuel your body, boost your energy, and rejuvenate your appearance. Whether you're looking to prevent the signs of aging, reverse the clock, or simply maintain your youthful glow, **The Quick And Easy Forever Strong Diet Cookbook** has you covered.

Our journey begins by exploring the science behind aging and nutrition, offering you insights into the incredible power of food to nurture and heal your body. We'll delve into the essential nutrients, antioxidants, and superfoods that can help turn back the hands of time.

But this cookbook is not just about theory. It's about practical, mouthwatering solutions that you can incorporate into your daily life. From rejuvenating breakfast smoothies to nutrient-rich main courses and delightful desserts that won't compromise your goals, we've created recipes that are as satisfying as they are healthful.

In addition to an array of delectable dishes, we'll provide you with tips, meal plans, and guidance to help you stay on track and create a sustainable, age-defying lifestyle. We believe that the journey to lasting youth is a holistic one, encompassing not only the foods we eat but also the way we think and live.

We invite you to embrace **The Quick And Easy Forever Strong Diet Cookbook** as your trusted companion on the path to vibrant health, lasting beauty, and unshakable confidence. It's time to reclaim your youth, one delectable dish at a time. So, let's dive in, savor the flavors of vitality, and uncover the secret to looking and feeling younger, forever.

CHAPTER 1: BREAKFAST DELIGHTS

A. ENERGIZING MORNING SMOOTHIES

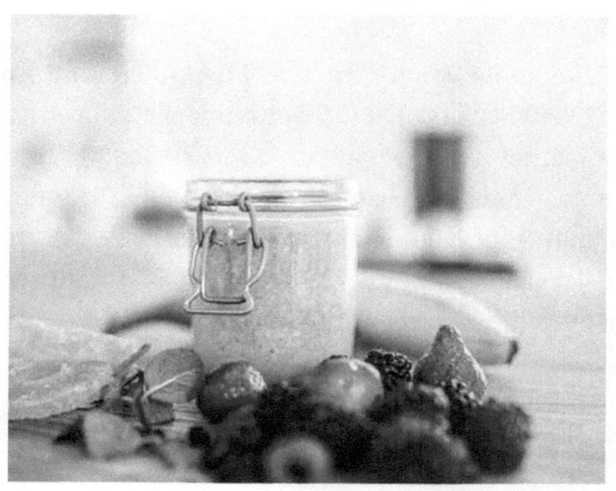

1. Green Goddess Glow Smoothie

Ingredients:

- 1 cup fresh spinach or kale
- 1/2 cucumber, peeled and chopped

- 1 green apple, cored and sliced
- 1/2 lemon, juiced
- 1 cup coconut water
- 1 tablespoon chia seeds
- Ice cubes (optional)

Instructions:

This recipe involves preparing spinach or kale, a cucumber, a green apple, a lemon, chia seeds, and a smoothie base. The spinach or kale is washed and patted dry, while the cucumber is chopped into small pieces for a refreshing and hydrating element. The green apple is sliced, leaving the skin on for added fiber and nutrients. The lemon juice is squeezed into a small bowl, ensuring the smoothie isn't overly tangy. Chia seeds are prepared by preparing a tablespoon of omega-3 fatty acids, fiber, and protein.

The spinach or kale is blended with the cucumber, apple, lemon juice, coconut water, and chia seeds. The apple adds natural sweetness to the earthy flavors of the greens, while the lemon juice enhances the overall flavor. The coconut water is hydrating and replenishes essential electrolytes, leaving the skin glowing. Chia seeds are sprinkled into the blender, providing a boost of healthy fats and fiber. Ice cubes can be added for extra cooling.

The smoothie is blended until a smooth, vibrant green consistency is achieved. The Green Goddess Glow Smoothie is a nutritional powerhouse that helps maintain youthful vitality and provides a refreshing drink for a day. Enjoy the vibrant green color and taste of this healthy smoothie.

2. Berry Blast Antioxidant Smoothie

Ingredients:

- 1 cup mixed berries (strawberries, blueberries, raspberries)
- 1/2 banana
- 1/2 cup Greek yogurt
- 1 tablespoon honey or agave nectar
- 1/2 cup almond milk
- 1 teaspoon flaxseed (optional)
- Ice cubes (optional)

Instructions:

To prepare a Berry Blast Antioxidant Smoothie, start by preparing mixed berries, such as strawberries, blueberries, and raspberries. Cut half of a banana into small slices for added sweetness. Measure 1/2 cup of Greek yogurt for protein and probiotics. Add honey or agave nectar to enhance sweetness. Add 1/2 cup of almond milk for a creamy base. Add 1 teaspoon of flaxseed for extra omega-3 fatty acids and fiber. Optionally, add ice cubes for extra coldness. Blend all ingredients until a vibrant purple or red hue is achieved. Serve and enjoy the refreshing, fruity flavors of this nutritional powerhouse, which supports overall health and radiates youthful vitality. Enjoy your day with this delicious and nutritious smoothie.

3. Tropical Turmeric Twist Smoothie

Ingredients:

- 1 cup frozen pineapple chunks
- 1/2 banana
- 1/2 teaspoon turmeric powder
- 1 tablespoon fresh ginger, grated
- 1 cup coconut milk
- 1 teaspoon honey or agave nectar (optional)
- Ice cubes (optional)

Instructions:

To prepare a tropical smoothie, blend frozen pineapple, banana, turmeric, fresh ginger, coconut milk, honey, ice cubes, and a touch of spiciness. Add 1 cup of frozen pineapple chunks for a refreshing twist, 1/2 teaspoon of turmeric powder for its anti-inflammatory properties, and 1 tablespoon of fresh ginger for its zesty spiciness. Add 1 cup of coconut milk for its tropical base and healthy fats. Optionally, add 1 teaspoon of honey or agave nectar for sweetness. If you prefer a chilled, frosty smoothie, add ice cubes. Blend all ingredients until smooth, which should take a minute or two. Serve and enjoy the tropical twist smoothie, which is not only delicious but also a nutritional powerhouse, thanks to the antioxidants in turmeric and the vitamins in the tropical fruit. This tropical twist supports your quest for lasting youth and vitality.

4. Chocolate Peanut Butter Power Smoothie

Ingredients:

- 1 ripe banana
- 2 tablespoons unsweetened cocoa powder
- 2 tablespoons natural peanut butter
- 1 cup unsweetened almond milk
- 1 teaspoon honey or agave nectar (optional)
- Ice cubes (optional)

Instructions:

To create a Chocolate Peanut Butter Power Smoothie, start by peeling and slicing a ripe banana for natural sweetness and creaminess. Add 2 tablespoons of unsweetened cocoa powder for a rich chocolatey flavor. Add 2 tablespoons of natural peanut butter for a creamy, nutty richness. Pour 1 cup of unsweetened almond milk for a smooth, dairy-free base. Optionally, add 1 teaspoon of honey or agave nectar for a touch of sweetness. If you prefer a colder, refreshing smoothie, add ice cubes. Blend all ingredients until a creamy and chocolatey delight is achieved, which should take a minute or two. Serve and enjoy the indulgent flavors of chocolate and peanut butter, providing protein and energy for a day of lasting youth and vitality.

5. Energizing Coffee-Infused Smoothie

Ingredients:

- 1 cup brewed coffee, cooled (you can use regular or decaffeinated coffee, based on your preference)
- 1/2 cup Greek yogurt
- 1 ripe banana
- 1-2 tablespoons almond butter
- 1 teaspoon honey or maple syrup (optional for added sweetness)
- Ice cubes (optional)
- 1/2 teaspoon cocoa powder (optional, for a hint of chocolate flavor)

Instructions:

The first step in making an energizing coffee-infused smoothie is to brew your favorite coffee and let it cool to room temperature. Before adding Greek yogurt for smoothness and an additional protein boost, prepare a banana for natural sweetness and a creamy texture. To add more protein and a nutty richness, add one or two tablespoons of almond butter. Maple syrup or honey can be used to provide optional sweetness. Add ice cubes for a refreshing smoothie. Add 1/2 teaspoon cocoa powder for a bit of chocolate flavor. Combine the chilled coffee with the other ingredients in the blender. Blend until smooth, being sure to fully incorporate all the ingredients. Serve and savor the revitalizing blend of creamy richness and coffee. This protein-rich smoothie with coffee infusion gives you a boost of energy to start the day. With this coffee-infused treat, enjoy your day!

6. Immune-Boosting Citrus Smoothie

Ingredients:

- 1 orange, peeled and segmented
- 1 grapefruit, peeled and segmented
- 1/2 cup Greek yogurt
- 1-2 tablespoons honey (adjust to taste)

- 1/2 cup coconut water
- Ice cubes (optional)

Instructions:

To make an Immune-Boosting Citrus Smoothie, peel and segment orange and grapefruit, remove seeds, and add Greek yogurt for creaminess and probiotics. Add honey, adjust sweetness, and add coconut water for a refreshing tropical base. Optional ice cubes can be added for extra coldness. Blend all ingredients until smooth, taking a minute or two. Serve and enjoy the refreshing citrus flavors in a glass, as this smoothie is not only delicious but also a nutritional powerhouse with vitamins and antioxidants. This citrus smoothie boosts the immune system and keeps you feeling your best. Enjoy your day with this zesty delight!

B. SUPERFOOD BREAKFAST BOWLS

1. Acai Berry Bliss Bowl

Ingredients:

For the Acai Bowl:

- 1 pack of frozen unsweetened acai berry puree (you can find these in the frozen section of health food stores or online)
- 1/2 banana
- 1/2 cup mixed berries (strawberries, blueberries, raspberries)
- 1/2 cup unsweetened almond milk (or your choice of milk)
- 1 tablespoon honey or agave nectar (optional, for added sweetness)

For Toppings (Customize to Your Liking):

- Sliced fresh berries (e.g., strawberries, blueberries, raspberries)
- Sliced banana
- Granola
- Chia seeds
- Shredded coconut
- Sliced almonds
- Honey drizzle

Instructions:

The frozen acai berry puree pack should first be prepared by briefly running it under warm water before adding it to an Acai Berry Bliss Bowl. Smooth and creamy texture is achieved by blending the acai pack, banana, mixed berries, unsweetened almond milk, and honey or agave nectar. As the acai base is blending, chop the bananas and fresh berries and arrange them in a chosen pattern, such as granola, chia seeds, shredded coconut, sliced almonds, and drizzled with honey. Transfer the pureed acai blend into a bowl and sprinkle or arrange the toppings on top in various patterns. Savor the mouthwatering blend of crunchy, sweet, and tangy tastes that is loaded with nutrients and antioxidants.

2. Chia Pudding Power Bowl

Ingredients:

For the Chia Pudding:
- 1/4 cup chia seeds
- 1 cup almond milk (or your choice of milk)
- 1/2 teaspoon vanilla extract
- 1 tablespoon honey or maple syrup (optional, for sweetness)

For Toppings (Customize to Your Liking):

- Sliced fresh fruit (e.g., berries, banana, kiwi)
- Nuts and seeds (e.g., almonds, pumpkin seeds)

- Shredded coconut
- Dried fruits (e.g., raisins, cranberries)
- A drizzle of honey or a dollop of Greek yogurt

Instructions:

To make a Chia Pudding Power Bowl, combine 1/4 cup of chia seeds, 1 cup of almond milk, 1/2 teaspoon of vanilla extract, and 1 tablespoon of honey or maple syrup in a bowl. Cover and let the mixture sit in the refrigerator for a few hours or overnight. While the chia pudding is setting, prepare desired toppings such as fresh fruits, nuts, seeds, shredded coconut, dried fruits, and honey or yogurt.

Assemble the Chia Pudding Bowl by removing it from the refrigerator and adding more milk if needed. Spoon the chia pudding into a bowl and arrange your desired toppings on top. For extra flavor and creaminess, drizzle honey or Greek yogurt on top. Enjoy your Chia Pudding Power Bowl, a nutritious and satisfying breakfast or snack packed with protein, fiber, and healthy fats.

3. Quinoa and Blueberry Breakfast Bowl

Ingredients:

For the Quinoa:
- 1/2 cup quinoa, rinsed
- 1 cup water
- 1/2 teaspoon vanilla extract
- 1/2 teaspoon ground cinnamon
- 1 tablespoon honey or maple syrup (optional, for sweetness)

For the Toppings (Customize to Your Liking):

- Fresh blueberries
- Sliced banana
- Chopped nuts (e.g., almonds, walnuts)
- Greek yogurt
- Drizzle of honey

Instructions:

Rinse the quinoa well then add water, vanilla essence, and ground cinnamon to make a Quinoa and Blueberry Breakfast Bowl. After bringing the mixture to a boil, lower the heat, cover it, and simmer it for fifteen minutes. Add some honey or maple syrup for sweetness, if you'd like. After cooking, let the quinoa cool slightly or chill it immediately in the refrigerator. As the quinoa cools, prepare the toppings by slicing a banana, rinsing fresh blueberries, chopping almonds, and preparing Greek yogurt and honey.

Spoon the cooked and slightly cooled quinoa over the base of the breakfast dish, then top with chopped almonds, sliced banana, and fresh blueberries. For richness and a hint of tang, add Greek yogurt. Pour honey on top if you'd like it to be sweeter.

Savor the satisfying and wholesome Quinoa and Blueberry Breakfast Bowl, which combines a tasty blend of crunchy almonds, creamy yogurt, sweet blueberries, and fluffy quinoa in a pleasant way.

4. Green Superfood Smoothie Bowl

Ingredients:

For the Green Smoothie Base:

- 1 cup fresh spinach or kale (or a combination of both)
- 1/2 banana
- 1/2 cup frozen mango chunks
- 1/2 cup frozen pineapple chunks
- 1/2 cup unsweetened almond milk (or your choice of milk)
- 1 tablespoon chia seeds
- 1 teaspoon honey or agave nectar (optional, for sweetness)

For Toppings (Customize to Your Liking):

- Sliced kiwi
- Fresh berries (e.g., strawberries, blueberries)
- Sliced banana
- Granola
- Chia seeds
- Shredded coconut
- Nuts or seeds (e.g., almonds, pumpkin seeds)
- A drizzle of honey

Instructions:

This recipe for a Green Superfood Smoothie Bowl involves blending spinach, kale, banana, frozen mango, and pineapple chunks in a blender for a vibrant green base. Add unsweetened almond milk for a smooth consistency, and add chia seeds for fiber and omega-3 fatty acids. If desired, add honey or agave nectar for a sweeter base. Blend until smooth, ensuring the mixture is thick enough to eat with a spoon.

While the base is blending, prepare desired toppings such as kiwi, fresh berries, banana, granola, chia seeds, shredded coconut, and nuts or seeds. Pour the smoothie base into a bowl, arrange the toppings creatively, and drizzle with honey for an extra touch of sweetness. Enjoy the nutritious and energizing Green Superfood Smoothie Bowl, packed with vitamins, minerals, and antioxidants, as a nutritious breakfast or snack to kickstart your day.

5. Spirulina Protein Bowl

Ingredients:

For the Spirulina Protein Bowl Base:

- 1 ripe banana
- 1/2 cup Greek yogurt
- 1 teaspoon spirulina powder
- 1 tablespoon honey or maple syrup (optional, for sweetness)
- 1/2 teaspoon vanilla extract
- A pinch of salt

For Toppings (Customize to Your Liking):

- Sliced fresh fruit (e.g., berries, kiwi, banana)
- Chopped nuts or seeds (e.g., almonds, chia seeds)
- Dried fruits (e.g., goji berries, raisins)
- Granola or muesli
- A drizzle of honey

Instructions:

To make a Spirulina Protein Bowl, blend 1 ripe banana, 1/2 cup of Greek yogurt, 1 teaspoon of spirulina powder, 1 tablespoon of honey or maple syrup, 1/2 teaspoon of vanilla extract, and a pinch of salt in a blender until smooth. This forms the base of the bowl. While the base is blending, prepare desired toppings such as fresh fruits, nuts or seeds, dried fruits, granola, and honey. Pour the green spirulina protein base into a bowl, arrange the toppings on top, and drizzle with honey for an extra touch of sweetness. Enjoy this visually striking, nutritious, and energizing bowl as a nutritious start to the day or a post-workout refuel.

6. Oat and Goji Berry Breakfast Bowl

Ingredients:

For the Oat and Goji Berry Base:

- 1/2 cup rolled oats
- 1 cup milk of your choice (e.g., almond milk, dairy milk)
- 1 tablespoon honey or maple syrup (optional, for sweetness)
- 1/4 teaspoon vanilla extract
- 2 tablespoons dried goji berries

For Toppings (Customize to Your Liking):

- Sliced fresh fruit (e.g., strawberries, banana, kiwi)
- Chopped nuts (e.g., almonds, walnuts)
- Seeds (e.g., chia seeds, flaxseeds)
- Dried coconut flakes
- A drizzle of honey

Instructions:

This recipe involves preparing the Oat and Goji Berry Base by combining rolled oats and milk in a saucepan. Cook the oats for 5-7 minutes, add honey or maple syrup, and vanilla extract for added sweetness. While the oats are simmering, prepare desired toppings such as fresh fruits, nuts, seeds, and dried coconut flakes.

Assemble the Breakfast Bowl by spooning the cooked oat and goji berry mixture into a bowl, arranging the toppings on top, and drizzling honey for an extra touch of sweetness. Enjoy this hearty and wholesome breakfast, packed with fiber, vitamins, and antioxidants, making it a nutritious way to start your day with a burst of energy. The recipe is a delicious and nutritious way to start your day.

C. ANTI-AGING OATMEAL VARIATIONS

1. Blueberry and Chia Seed Oatmeal

Ingredients:

- 1/2 cup rolled oats
- 1 cup milk (dairy, almond, or your choice)
- 1/2 cup fresh blueberries
- 1 tablespoon chia seeds
- 1 tablespoon honey or maple syrup (optional, for sweetness)
- 1/2 teaspoon vanilla extract
- A pinch of salt

Instructions:

This recipe involves preparing rolled oats by boiling one cup of milk and half a cup of rolled oats in a pot over medium heat. The oats should be simmered for 5 to 7 minutes until desired thickness is achieved. To add flavor, add 1/2 cup of fresh blueberries, 1 tablespoon of chia seeds, 1 tablespoon of honey or maple syrup, 1/2 teaspoon of vanilla essence, and a dash of salt to the cooked oats. Stir everything together well, as the blueberries will soften and impart their flavor due to the heat. Transfer the oats to a bowl and enjoy the creamy, nutty chia seed and sweet blueberry blend. This healthy meal provides fiber, antioxidants, and other nutrients to start your day.

2. Nutty Banana Oatmeal

Ingredients:

- 1/2 cup rolled oats
- 1 cup milk (dairy, almond, or your choice)
- 1 ripe banana, sliced
- 1 tablespoon chopped nuts (e.g., almonds, walnuts)
- 1 tablespoon honey or maple syrup (optional, for sweetness)
- 1/2 teaspoon vanilla extract
- A pinch of cinnamon (optional)
- A pinch of salt

Instructions:

This recipe involves preparing rolled oats by adding milk and rolled oats to a pot and boiling over medium heat. The oats should be simmered for 5 to 7 minutes until desired thickness is achieved. After cooking, add a ripe banana, chopped nuts, honey or maple syrup, vanilla essence, salt, and cinnamon. Stir everything together well, as the banana will soften and give the oats a sweeter taste due to the heat. Serve the crunchy banana oats in a bowl, enjoying the sweet banana, crunch, and creamy oats. This meal is a great way to start the day and is full of fiber, potassium, and other essential minerals. Feel free to add additional toppings or spices to the oatmeal.

3. Pumpkin Pie Spice Oatmeal

Ingredients:

- 1/2 cup rolled oats
- 1 cup milk (dairy, almond, or your choice)
- 1/4 cup canned pumpkin puree
- 1 tablespoon maple syrup or honey (adjust to taste)
- 1/2 teaspoon pumpkin pie spice (a blend of cinnamon, nutmeg, allspice, and cloves)
- 1/2 teaspoon vanilla extract
- A pinch of salt
- Chopped nuts (e.g., pecans, walnuts) and dried cranberries for topping (optional)

Instructions:

This recipe involves preparing rolled oats by adding milk and rolled oats to a pot and boiling over medium heat. The oats should be steamed for 5 to 7 minutes until desired thickness is achieved. Next, add canned pumpkin puree, maple syrup, pumpkin pie spice, vanilla essence, and salt. Stir and warm the oatmeal for two to three minutes to combine flavors. Optional toppings include chopped nuts and dried cranberries for texture and taste. The oatmeal can be served with a bowl of sweet pumpkin, creamy oats, and pumpkin pie spice, making it a nutritious and fiber-rich meal perfect for chilly mornings. The recipe can be personalized by adding more toppings or a dash of extra spice. Enjoy the taste of this delicious oatmeal with Pumpkin Pie Spice!

4. Cinnamon Apple Oatmeal

Ingredients:

- 1/2 cup rolled oats
- 1 cup milk (dairy, almond, or your choice)
- 1 medium apple, peeled, cored, and diced
- 1 tablespoon honey or maple syrup (adjust to taste)
- 1/2 teaspoon ground cinnamon
- A pinch of salt
- Chopped nuts (e.g., walnuts, pecans) and raisins for topping (optional)

Instructions:

This recipe involves preparing rolled oats by adding milk and rolled oats to a pot and boiling over medium heat. The oats should be simmered for 5 to 7 minutes until desired thickness is achieved. After cooking, add diced apples, cinnamon, honey, and salt to the oatmeal. Stir and warm the mixture, allowing the apple to soften for two to three minutes. Optional toppings include chopped nuts or raisins for extra texture. The oatmeal is filling, tasty, and ideal for a chilly morning. It is rich in fiber, vitamins, and natural sweetness, making it an ideal breakfast option. The dish can be served in a dish, providing a cozy and satisfying experience.

5. *Almond Joy Oatmeal*

Ingredients:

- 1/2 cup rolled oats
- 1 cup milk (dairy, almond, or your choice)
- 2 tablespoons unsweetened shredded coconut
- 2 tablespoons chopped almonds
- 2 tablespoons chocolate chips or chocolate chunks (dark or milk chocolate, as per your preference)
- 1-2 tablespoons honey or maple syrup (adjust to taste)
- A pinch of salt

Instructions:

This recipe involves preparing rolled oats by boiling one cup of milk and half a cup of rolled oats in a pot over medium heat. The oats should be simmered for 5 to 7 minutes until desired thickness is achieved. After cooking, add chopped almonds and unsweetened shredded coconut, stirring well. Add two teaspoons of chocolate chunks or chips, stirring until they melt and give the oats a delicious chocolate taste. To make the oats sweeter, add 1-2 tablespoons of honey or maple syrup, or more to taste, and sprinkle a little salt. Stir everything together well, and the oats should be creamy, chocolaty, and almond-coconut. Transfer the Almond Joy oats into a bowl and enjoy the mouthwatering blend of chocolate, coconut, almonds, and creamy oats. This decadent breakfast resembles the popular Almond Joy candy bar.

6. Cranberry Orange Oatmeal

Ingredients:

- 1/2 cup rolled oats
- 1 cup milk (dairy, almond, or your choice)
- 1/4 cup dried cranberries
- Zest and juice of 1 orange

- 1-2 tablespoons honey or maple syrup (adjust to taste)
- A pinch of salt
- Sliced almonds or chopped walnuts for topping (optional)

Instructions:

This recipe involves preparing rolled oats by boiling one cup of milk and half a cup of rolled oats over medium heat. The oats should be simmered for 5 to 7 minutes until desired thickness is achieved. After cooking, add 1/4 cup of dried cranberries and one orange's zest to the oats, bringing the taste of fresh orange to the oats. To sweeten the oats, add 1-2 teaspoons of maple syrup or honey, and stir the oats to include all ingredients. A small teaspoon of salt is added for flavor. Optional toppings like chopped walnuts or sliced almonds can add texture and nutty taste. The Cranberry Orange Oatmeal is a delicious, fruity meal that will brighten your morning.

D. PROTEIN-PACKED PANCAKES AND WAFFLES

1. *Classic Protein Pancakes*

Ingredients:

- 1 cup all-purpose flour
- 2 tablespoons protein powder (vanilla or unflavored)
- 2 tablespoons granulated sugar
- 1 teaspoon baking powder
- 1/2 teaspoon baking soda
- 1/4 teaspoon salt
- 1 cup buttermilk
- 1 large egg
- 2 tablespoons melted butter or vegetable oil
- 1 teaspoon vanilla extract

Instructions:

Preheat a non-stick pan or griddle to medium heat and lightly oil the surface. Mix dry ingredients such as flour, protein powder, sugar, baking powder, baking soda, and salt in a mixing bowl. Prepare wet ingredients by mixing egg, buttermilk, melted butter, and vanilla essence. Transfer the liquid components into the dry ingredients and mix until barely incorporated.

Prepare the pancakes by transferring 1/4 cup of batter onto a hot griddle or skillet and simmering for two to three minutes. Flip the pancakes over and cook for an additional two to three minutes until well cooked and golden brown on both sides.

Serve the pancakes warm and top with Greek yogurt, fresh fruit, or maple syrup. You can adjust the amount of sugar and protein powder to suit your taste and dietary requirements. These high-protein pancakes provide a satisfying and nourishing meal to start the day.

2. Banana Nut Protein Waffles

Ingredients:

- 1 cup all-purpose flour
- 1/2 cup protein powder (vanilla or unflavored)
- 1 tablespoon granulated sugar
- 1 teaspoon baking powder
- 1/2 teaspoon baking soda
- 1/4 teaspoon salt
- 2 ripe bananas, mashed
- 2 large eggs
- 1 cup buttermilk
- 1/4 cup melted butter or vegetable oil
- 1/2 cup chopped walnuts or pecans
- 1 teaspoon vanilla extract

Instructions:

To make Banana Nut Protein Waffles, follow the manufacturer's instructions and preheat your waffle iron. Combine dry ingredients like flour, protein powder, sugar, baking powder, baking soda, and salt in a mixing dish. Mash two ripe bananas, buttermilk, oil, vanilla extract, and eggs in a separate basin. Transfer the liquid mixture to the dry ingredients and mix until barely incorporated. Gently mix 1/2 cup of chopped pecans or walnuts into the waffle mixture.

Place the batter onto the hot waffle iron and cook until crisp and golden brown. If necessary, lightly lubricate the iron with oil or cooking spray. Pour the batter onto the iron and cook until crisp and golden brown.

Serve the waffles with toppings like sliced bananas, almonds, Greek yogurt, honey, or maple syrup. Enjoy the protein-rich and delicious Banana Nut Protein Waffles for breakfast, which can be easily modified to suit your taste by changing the protein powder flavor and sugar amount. These waffles are a delicious and filling breakfast that will start your day.

3. Berry Bliss Protein Pancakes

Ingredients:

- 1 cup all-purpose flour
- 1/2 cup protein powder (vanilla or berry-flavored)
- 2 tablespoons granulated sugar
- 1 teaspoon baking powder
- 1/2 teaspoon baking soda
- 1/4 teaspoon salt
- 1 cup buttermilk
- 1 large egg
- 2 tablespoons melted butter or vegetable oil
- 1 teaspoon vanilla extract
- 1/2 cup mixed berries (e.g., strawberries, blueberries, raspberries)

Instructions:

Firstly, preheat a non-stick pan or griddle to medium heat and lightly oil the surface. Combine dry ingredients such as flour, protein powder, sugar, baking powder, baking soda, and salt in a mixing dish. Prepare wet ingredients by mixing egg, buttermilk, butter or vegetable oil, and vanilla essence. Transfer the liquid components into the dry ingredients and mix until barely incorporated.

Incorporate mixed berries into the pancake mixture, saving some for topping. Prepare the pancakes by transferring 1/4 cup of batter onto a hot griddle or skillet and simmering for two to three minutes. Flip the pancakes over and cook for an additional two to three minutes until well cooked and golden brown on both sides.

Serve the pancakes warm and enjoy the homemade protein-rich pancakes flavored with a variety of berries. Feel free to add your preferred berry varieties and adjust the sugar amount to suit your nutritional needs. These Berry Bliss Protein Pancakes are a tasty and healthy way to start the day.

4. Chocolate Protein Waffles

Ingredients:

- 1 cup all-purpose flour
- 1/2 cup protein powder (chocolate-flavored)
- 2 tablespoons unsweetened cocoa powder
- 2 tablespoons granulated sugar
- 1 teaspoon baking powder
- 1/2 teaspoon baking soda
- 1/4 teaspoon salt
- 1 cup buttermilk
- 1 large egg
- 2 tablespoons melted butter or vegetable oil
- 1/2 teaspoon vanilla extract
- 1/4 cup chocolate chips (optional)

- Whipped cream and fresh berries for topping (optional)

Instructions:

To make chocolate protein waffles, follow the manufacturer's instructions and preheat your waffle iron. Combine dry ingredients like flour, protein powder, unsweetened cocoa powder, sugar, baking powder, baking soda, and salt in a mixing bowl. Prepare wet ingredients by mixing an egg, buttermilk, melted butter, and vanilla essence. Transfer the liquid components into the dry ingredients and mix until barely incorporated. Optionally, add 1/4 cup of chocolate chips to the batter.

Place the batter on the hot waffle iron and cook according to the manufacturer's instructions. Once crispy and rich in chocolate, close the iron and cook. Serve the waffles and top them with fresh berries and whipped cream. Enjoy the delicious, high-protein, chocolate-flavored breakfast to start the day. You can add additional toppings like more chocolate chips, chopped nuts, or a drizzle of chocolate syrup to suit your taste. Enjoy your freshly cooked chocolate protein waffles, providing a delicious, high-protein, and chocolate-flavored breakfast to start the day.

5. Peanut Butter Protein Pancakes

Ingredients:

- 1 cup all-purpose flour
- 1/2 cup protein powder (vanilla or peanut butter flavored)
- 2 tablespoons granulated sugar
- 1 teaspoon baking powder
- 1/2 teaspoon baking soda
- 1/4 teaspoon salt
- 1 cup buttermilk
- 1/4 cup creamy peanut butter
- 1 large egg
- 2 tablespoons melted butter or vegetable oil
- 1 teaspoon vanilla extract

Instructions:

Preheat a non-stick pan or griddle to medium heat and lightly oil the surface. Combine dry ingredients such as flour, protein powder, sugar, baking powder, baking soda, and salt in a mixing dish. Prepare wet ingredients by mixing buttermilk, egg, butter or vegetable oil, vanilla extract, and creamy peanut butter in a separate dish. Transfer the liquid components into the dry ingredients and mix until barely incorporated.

Prepare the pancakes by transferring 1/4 cup of batter onto a hot griddle or skillet and simmering for two to three minutes. Flip the pancakes over and cook for an additional two to three minutes until well cooked and golden brown on both sides. Set the pancakes aside to stay warm and serve with desired toppings like chopped peanuts, sliced bananas, or honey or maple syrup. Enjoy the freshly prepared, high-protein pancakes with a delectable peanut butter twist, and add extra toppings or spices to your liking. A satisfying and high-protein meal is what these Peanut Butter Protein Pancakes are all about.

6. Almond Joy Protein Waffles

Ingredients:

- 1 cup all-purpose flour
- 1/2 cup protein powder (chocolate or vanilla flavored)
- 2 tablespoons unsweetened cocoa powder
- 2 tablespoons granulated sugar
- 1 teaspoon baking powder
- 1/2 teaspoon baking soda
- 1/4 teaspoon salt
- 1 cup buttermilk
- 1/4 cup melted butter or vegetable oil

- 1 large egg
- 1/2 teaspoon almond extract
- 1/4 cup shredded coconut
- 1/4 cup chopped almonds
- 1/4 cup chocolate chips (optional)
- Whipped cream and additional almonds for topping (optional)

Instructions:

To make Almond Joy protein waffles, follow the manufacturer's instructions to preheat your waffle iron and mix dry ingredients in a mixing dish. Prepare wet ingredients by mixing buttermilk, melted butter, egg, and almond essence. Transfer the liquid components into the dry ingredients and mix until barely incorporated. Add chocolate chips, chopped almonds, and shredded coconut to the batter.

Place the batter on the hot waffle iron and cook according to the manufacturer's directions. Once crispy and smelling rich, close the iron and cook. Serve the waffles and maintain their temperature. Add more toppings like chopped almonds, whipped cream, or other desired toppings.

These homemade protein waffles provide a delicious, high-protein, and decadent breakfast to start the day. You can customize the flavor of the protein powder and sugar amount to suit your tastes. Enjoy your homemade protein waffles, Almond Joy! These waffles provide a delicious, high-protein, and decadent breakfast to start the day.

CHAPTER 2: WHOLESOME SOUPS AND SALADS

A. GARDEN-FRESH SALAD CREATIONS

1. *Mediterranean Chickpea Salad*

Ingredients:

For the Salad:

- 2 cans (15 oz each) of chickpeas, drained and rinsed
- 1 cup cherry tomatoes, halved
- 1 cucumber, diced
- 1 red onion, finely chopped
- 1/2 cup Kalamata olives, pitted and sliced
- 1/2 cup crumbled feta cheese
- 1/4 cup fresh parsley, chopped

- 1/4 cup fresh mint, chopped

For the Dressing:

- 1/4 cup extra-virgin olive oil
- 3 tablespoons lemon juice
- 2 cloves garlic, minced
- 1 teaspoon dried oregano
- Salt and pepper to taste

Instructions:

This recipe involves making a Mediterranean Chickpea Salad. First, mix extra virgin olive oil, lemon juice, dried oregano, minced garlic, salt, and pepper in a bowl. Then, combine diced cucumber, sliced red onion, feta cheese, crumbled feta cheese, fresh parsley, and mint in a large salad dish. Drizzle the dressing over the salad components, ensuring it coats everything evenly. Chill the salad in the refrigerator for about half an hour to allow flavors to blend. After cooling, serve the salad on a tray or in separate bowls, garnishing with more parsley or mint if desired. This light and revitalizing salad is perfect for a nutritious lunch or supper, and is also a great addition to potlucks and picnics.

2. Strawberry Spinach Salad with Balsamic Vinaigrette

Ingredients:

For the Salad:

- 6 cups fresh baby spinach leaves
- 2 cups fresh strawberries, hulled and sliced
- 1/2 cup crumbled feta cheese
- 1/4 cup red onion, thinly sliced
- 1/4 cup candied pecans or sliced almonds (optional for added crunch)

For the Balsamic Vinaigrette:

- 1/4 cup extra-virgin olive oil
- 2 tablespoons balsamic vinegar
- 1 teaspoon Dijon mustard
- 1 clove garlic, minced
- 1 teaspoon honey (adjust to taste)
- Salt and pepper to taste

Instructions:

Prepare a balsamic vinaigrette by combining extra virgin olive oil, honey, balsamic vinegar, Dijon mustard, minced garlic, salt, and pepper. Adjust the sweetness if needed. Combine fresh baby spinach leaves, sliced strawberries, crumbled feta cheese, thinly sliced red onion, and candied nuts or almonds in a large salad dish. Pour the dressing over the salad, tossing gently to ensure even coverage. Refrigerate for ten to fifteen minutes to allow flavors to combine. Serve the salad after cooling and settling. Enjoy this tasty and revitalizing meal that combines the tartness of the vinaigrette with the sweetness of the strawberries. This salad is a great complement to any dinner, especially when strawberries are in season. Enjoy it as a light and healthy main course or side dish.

3. Asian-Inspired Cucumber and Sesame Salad

Ingredients:

For the Salad:

- 2 large cucumbers, thinly sliced
- 1 medium carrot, julienned
- 2 green onions, finely chopped
- 2 tablespoons sesame seeds, toasted
- Fresh cilantro leaves, for garnish
- Red chili flakes, for a spicy kick (optional)

For the Dressing:

- 3 tablespoons soy sauce
- 2 tablespoons rice vinegar
- 1 tablespoon sesame oil

- 1 tablespoon honey or brown sugar
- 1 clove garlic, minced
- 1 teaspoon fresh ginger, grated
- Salt and pepper, to taste

Instructions:

This recipe for an Asian-inspired cucumber and sesame salad involves preparing a dressing by mixing soy sauce, rice vinegar, sesame oil, honey, grated ginger, chopped garlic, and salt & pepper. The vegetables are finely cut, thinly sliced, and julienned. The salad ingredients are combined in a large mixing dish, and toasted sesame seeds are added for a crunch and nutty taste. The dressing is then dripped over the vegetables, with a hint of red chili flakes added for heat. The salad is left to chill and marinate for 15 to 20 minutes, allowing flavors to combine. Fresh cilantro leaves are sprinkled over the salad just before serving. This salad can be served as a light appetizer or a cool side dish, making it an ideal choice for barbecues and dinners with Asian influences. The combination of crisp cucumbers, crunchy sesame seeds, and a tasty dressing creates a filling and refreshing Asian-inspired meal.

4. Caprese Salad with Heirloom Tomatoes and Fresh Basil

Ingredients:

For the Salad:

- 4 large heirloom tomatoes, sliced into 1/4-inch rounds
- 8 ounces fresh mozzarella cheese, sliced into 1/4-inch rounds
- Fresh basil leaves
- Extra-virgin olive oil
- Balsamic glaze (or balsamic reduction)
- Salt and freshly ground black pepper, to taste

For the Balsamic Glaze:

- 1/2 cup balsamic vinegar
- 2 tablespoons honey or brown sugar

Instructions:

To prepare a caprese salad, combine honey and balsamic vinegar in a small pot over medium heat. Simmer the mixture for 10 to 15 minutes over low heat, then let it cool. Compose the salad by placing fresh mozzarella and heirloom tomato slices in an alternating pattern on a large serving plate. Drizzle with extra virgin olive oil and pour the chilled balsamic glaze over the salad for a tart and sweet taste. Season and serve with freshly ground black pepper and a dash of salt to taste. Garnish with more basil leaves to enhance the salad's scent and appearance. Serve the caprese salad as a traditional starter or side dish, topped with fresh basil and heirloom tomatoes. This ageless staple is easy to make and has a striking presentation and flavor. Enjoy the flavors and colors of heirloom tomatoes and the fresh, fragrant basil.

5. Grilled Peach and Arugula Salad with Honey-Dijon Dressing

Ingredients:

For the Salad:

- 4 ripe peaches, halved and pitted
- 8 cups fresh arugula
- 1/2 cup crumbled goat cheese
- 1/4 cup candied pecans, roughly chopped
- 1/4 cup red onion, thinly sliced
- Olive oil for grilling

For the Honey-Dijon Dressing:

- 3 tablespoons extra-virgin olive oil
- 1 tablespoon balsamic vinegar
- 1 tablespoon honey

- 1 teaspoon Dijon mustard
- Salt and freshly ground black pepper, to taste

Instructions:

In this recipe, extra-virgin olive oil, balsamic vinegar, honey, Dijon mustard, salt, and freshly ground black pepper are whisked together to make a Honey-Dijon Dressing. To keep the peaches from sticking, gently spray them with olive oil before grilling them over medium-high heat. After that, create the salad by adding grilled peach halves and fresh arugula to the top. Crushed goat cheese, candied walnuts, and finely sliced red onion are some of the toppings. The honey-Dijon dressing offers the ideal ratio of tart and sweet tastes. Next, add salt and freshly ground black pepper to taste while seasoning the salad. This meal is a delicious and sophisticated take on a summer salad, combining the refreshing bite of arugula with the sweetness of grilled peaches.

This salad is a great way to enjoy the smoky goodness of grilled peaches, the peppery notes of arugula, and the sweetness of the honey-Dijon dressing.

6. Roasted Beet and Goat Cheese Salad with Candied Pecans

50

Ingredients:

For the Salad:

- 4 medium beets (a mix of red and golden), peeled and cut into 1-inch chunks
- 4 cups mixed salad greens (e.g., arugula, baby spinach, or spring mix)
- 4 ounces goat cheese, crumbled
- 1/2 cup candied pecans, roughly chopped
- 1/4 cup red onion, thinly sliced

For the Candied Pecans:

- 1 cup pecan halves
- 1/4 cup granulated sugar
- 1 tablespoon unsalted butter
- A pinch of salt

For the Balsamic Vinaigrette:

- 3 tablespoons extra-virgin olive oil
- 2 tablespoons balsamic vinegar
- 1 teaspoon honey
- 1/2 teaspoon Dijon mustard
- Salt and freshly ground black pepper, to taste

Instructions:

For the Candied Pecans:

In a pan set over medium heat, melt unsalted butter. Spread butter over pecan halves, season with salt and granulated sugar, and cook for 5 to 7 minutes, or until caramelized. Take off the heat and place on parchment paper to cool. Roughly slice the candied pecans when they have cooled. Take caution not to burn them.

For the Salad:

Preheat the oven to 400°F or 200°C. Place beetroot on a baking sheet, cover with olive oil, and season with salt and pepper. Roast for 30-40 minutes until soft and easily punctured. Cool and serve with candied pecans, red onion, goat cheese, mixed salad greens, and roasted beets in a large salad dish.

For the Balsamic Vinaigrette:

Whisk together extra-virgin olive oil, balsamic vinegar, honey, Dijon mustard, salt, and black pepper in a bowl. Drizzle the balsamic vinaigrette over the salad and gently toss to coat. Serve the Roasted Beet and Goat Cheese Salad with Candied Pecans as a vibrant and delicious dish, combining the earthy sweetness of beets with the creaminess of goat cheese, the crunch of candied pecans, and the tangy balsamic vinaigrette.

7. Quinoa and Roasted Vegetable Salad with Lemon-Herb Dressing

Ingredients:

For the Salad:

- 1 cup quinoa, rinsed and cooked according to package instructions
- 2 cups mixed roasted vegetables (e.g., bell peppers, zucchini, cherry tomatoes, red onion)
- 1/4 cup crumbled feta cheese
- 1/4 cup fresh basil leaves, torn
- 1/4 cup fresh parsley, chopped
- 2 tablespoons pine nuts, toasted

For the Lemon-Herb Dressing:

- 1/4 cup extra-virgin olive oil
- Zest and juice of 1 lemon
- 1 clove garlic, minced
- 1 tablespoon fresh basil, finely chopped
- 1 tablespoon fresh parsley, finely chopped
- Salt and freshly ground black pepper, to taste

Instructions:

For the Salad:

Preheat the oven to 400°F or 200°C. Prepare the quinoa and let it cool. Roast the mixed roasted veggies with olive oil, salt, and pepper for 20-25 minutes until soft and caramelizing. Remove from the oven and let them cool. Combine the cooked quinoa, roasted veggies, feta cheese crumbles, parsley, basil leaves, and pine nuts in a large salad dish.

For the Lemon-Herb Dressing:

In a small bowl, combine extra virgin olive oil, lemon zest, juice, minced garlic, parsley, basil, salt, and ground black pepper. Add the salad to the bowl and drizzle with the lemon-herb dressing. Gently toss the salad to ensure it is evenly distributed. This delectable Quinoa and Roasted Vegetable Salad with Lemon-Herb Dressing is an ideal combination of quinoa, roasted vegetables, fresh herbs, and the dressing's tangy taste. Enjoy it as a side dish or a healthy meal on its own.

8. Watermelon and Feta Salad with Mint and a Balsamic Glaze

Ingredients:

For the Salad:

- 4 cups cubed seedless watermelon
- 1 cup crumbled feta cheese
- Fresh mint leaves, torn or chopped
- 1/4 red onion, thinly sliced

For the Balsamic Glaze:

- 1/2 cup balsamic vinegar
- 2 tablespoons honey or brown sugar

Instructions:

For the Balsamic Glaze:

Combine balsamic vinegar and honey in a small saucepan over medium heat. Reduce heat and let it simmer for 10-15 minutes until the mixture has reduced by half and thickened to a syrupy consistency. Remove from heat and let it cool.

For the Salad:

Crumble feta cheese and diced, seedless watermelon together in a large salad dish. Toss gently to combine ingredients; for a tart and sweet taste, sprinkle with cooled balsamic glaze. Garnish with thinly sliced red onion and add fresh mint leaves for color and flavor. This meal is visually beautiful as it mixes the creamy feta, fragrant mint, and balsamic glaze with the sweetness of watermelon.

Enjoy this salad as a delightful and elegant appetizer or side dish.

B. IMMUNE-BOOSTING SOUP RECIPES

1. Chicken and Vegetable Soup

Ingredients:

For the Soup:

- 1 pound boneless, skinless chicken breasts or thighs, cut into bite-sized pieces
- 1 onion, finely chopped
- 2 carrots, peeled and sliced
- 2 celery stalks, sliced
- 2 cloves garlic, minced

- 8 cups chicken broth (homemade or low-sodium store-bought)
- 1 cup green beans, trimmed and chopped
- 1 cup corn kernels (fresh, frozen, or canned)
- 1 cup peas (fresh or frozen)
- 1 bay leaf
- 1 teaspoon dried thyme
- Salt and pepper, to taste
- Olive oil for sautéing

For Garnish:

- Fresh parsley, chopped

Instructions:

In a large pot or Dutch oven, heat olive oil over medium-high heat and sauté onion, carrots, celery, minced garlic, chicken pieces, chicken broth, bay leaf, and dried thyme. Bring the soup to a boil, reduce heat to low, cover, and simmer for 20-25 minutes until chicken is fully cooked and vegetables are tender. Stir in green beans, corn, and peas and simmer for an additional 5-7 minutes. Season the soup with salt and pepper to taste, adjusting the salt based on personal preference and chicken broth's saltiness. Remove the bay leaf from the soup. Ladle the Chicken and Vegetable Soup into bowls, garnish with fresh parsley, and serve hot. This comforting and immune-boosting soup is packed with nutrients, protein, and flavor, making it a perfect choice for a hearty and healthy meal. Customize the soup by adding spinach, kale, or lemon juice for extra zest.

2. *Turmeric and Ginger Carrot Soup*

Ingredients:

For the Soup:

- 1 pound carrots, peeled and sliced
- 1 onion, chopped
- 2 cloves garlic, minced
- 1-inch piece of fresh ginger, peeled and grated
- 1 teaspoon ground turmeric
- 4 cups vegetable broth (homemade or store-bought)
- 1 can (14 ounces) of coconut milk
- 2 tablespoons olive oil
- Salt and pepper, to taste

For Garnish:

- Fresh cilantro, chopped
- Greek yogurt or coconut yogurt (optional)

Instructions:

In a large pot, heat olive oil over medium heat and sauté chopped onion, minced garlic, and grated ginger. Stir in ground turmeric, coating the ingredients. Add sliced carrots and cook for another 5 minutes. Pour in vegetable broth and bring to a boil. Reduce heat, cover, and simmer for 20-25 minutes until carrots are tender. Puree the soup using an immersion or regular blender. Return the soup to the pot and stir in coconut milk. Heat gently over low heat, not boiling. Season with salt and pepper to taste. Garnish with fresh cilantro and add Greek or coconut yogurt if desired. Enjoy this immune-boosting soup, perfect for any season, packed with anti-inflammatory ingredients known for their immune-boosting properties. This soup is not only delicious but also packed with anti-inflammatory properties.

3. Spinach and White Bean Soup

Ingredients:

For the Soup:

- 2 tablespoons olive oil
- 1 onion, finely chopped
- 2 cloves garlic, minced
- 2 carrots, diced
- 2 celery stalks, diced

- 1 can (15 ounces) white beans (cannellini or navy), drained and rinsed
- 6 cups vegetable broth (homemade or store-bought)
- 1 bay leaf
- 1 teaspoon dried thyme
- 4 cups fresh spinach, chopped
- Salt and pepper, to taste

For Garnish:

- Grated Parmesan cheese (optional)
- Fresh basil leaves, torn

Instructions:

In a large soup pot, sauté onion, garlic, carrots, and celery in olive oil for 5 minutes. Add white beans and cook for 2 minutes. Pour vegetable broth, bay leaf, and dried thyme, and bring to a gentle boil. Reduce heat, cover, and simmer for 20-25 minutes. Add spinach and cook for 2-3 minutes. Season with salt and pepper, then remove bay leaf. Ladle the soup into bowls, garnish with grated Parmesan cheese and fresh basil leaves. Garnish with grated Parmesan cheese if desired and add fresh basil leaves for extra flavor. Enjoy this nourishing and immune-boosting Spinach and White Bean Soup, which combines the goodness of white beans and vibrant spinach in a flavorful broth. Customize the soup with other vegetables or herbs, such as diced tomatoes or lemon juice.

4. Miso Soup with Shiitake Mushrooms

Ingredients:

For the Soup:

- 4 cups water
- 4 cups vegetable broth (homemade or store-bought)
- 1 cup shiitake mushrooms, sliced
- 1/2 cup sliced green onions (scallions)
- 1/4 cup miso paste (white or red, based on your preference)
- 1/2 cup tofu, cubed
- 1 sheet of nori (seaweed), cut into thin strips
- 1 teaspoon sesame oil
- 1 teaspoon soy sauce (optional, for added depth of flavor)
- Salt and pepper, to taste

For Garnish:

- Fresh cilantro leaves
- Sesame seeds

Instructions:

In a large pot, bring water and vegetable broth to a gentle boil. Add sliced shiitake mushrooms and green onions, reduce heat, and let the soup simmer for 5-7 minutes. Dilute the miso paste with hot broth to make it easier to incorporate. Stir the diluted miso paste into the soup, avoiding boiling to maintain flavor. Add cubed tofu and simmer for 2-3 minutes. Season with sesame oil and soy sauce, adjust seasoning with salt and pepper. Remove the soup from heat and discard the nori sheet. Ladle the Miso Soup with Shiitake Mushrooms into bowls, garnish with fresh cilantro leaves and sesame seeds, and serve hot. This comforting and immune-boosting soup combines the umami of miso with the earthy richness of shiitake mushrooms. It is rich in probiotics and antioxidants, making it an excellent choice for supporting the immune system.

5. *Lentil and Kale Soup*

Ingredients:

For the Soup:

- 1 cup green or brown lentils, rinsed and drained
- 1 onion, chopped

- 2 carrots, diced
- 2 celery stalks, diced
- 3 cloves garlic, minced
- 1 can (14 ounces) diced tomatoes
- 4 cups vegetable broth (homemade or store-bought)
- 4 cups water
- 4 cups fresh kale, stems removed and leaves chopped
- 1 teaspoon ground cumin
- 1 teaspoon ground coriander
- 1/2 teaspoon smoked paprika
- Salt and pepper, to taste
- Olive oil for sautéing

For Garnish:

- Fresh lemon wedges
- Fresh parsley, chopped

Instructions:

In a large pot, sauté onion, carrots, celery, garlic, cumin, coriander, and smoked paprika until softened. Add lentils, tomatoes, vegetable broth, and water, bring to a boil, reduce heat, cover, and simmer for 25-30 minutes until lentils are tender. Stir in chopped kale and simmer for an additional 5-7 minutes until wilted and tender. Season with salt and pepper to taste. Ladle the soup into bowls, garnish with lemon wedges and parsley, and serve hot. This hearty and immune-boosting dish combines lentils' richness with the vibrant green goodness of kale. Customize the soup with other vegetables or herbs, such as adding lemon juice for a zesty kick. Enjoy this nutritious and comforting dish.

6. Garlic and Lemon Chicken Soup

Ingredients:

For the Soup:

- 4 boneless, skinless chicken breasts, cut into bite-sized pieces
- 1 onion, finely chopped
- 4 cloves garlic, minced
- 4 cups chicken broth (homemade or store-bought)
- 4 cups water
- Juice of 2 lemons
- 1 teaspoon dried thyme
- 1 teaspoon dried oregano
- Salt and pepper, to taste
- Olive oil for sautéing

For Garnish:

- Fresh parsley, chopped
- Lemon wedges

Instructions:

In a large pot, sauté onion, minced garlic, and bite-sized chicken until translucent. Add chicken broth, water, dried thyme, and oregano, bring to a gentle boil, reduce heat, cover, and simmer for 20-25 minutes until fully cooked and tender. Add lemon juice for a bright, tangy flavor. Season with salt and pepper to taste. Ladle the soup into bowls, garnish with fresh parsley, and serve with lemon wedges. This soothing and immune-boosting soup combines the rich flavor of chicken with the zesty kick of lemon and aromatic herbs. Customize the soup with other herbs or spices, such as adding red pepper flakes for a hint of heat. Enjoy this soothing and immune-boosting soup.

7. Tomato Basil Soup with Immune-Boosting Herbs

Ingredients:

For the Soup:

- 2 tablespoons olive oil
- 1 onion, chopped

- 2 cloves garlic, minced
- 2 cans (28 ounces each) whole tomatoes
- 4 cups vegetable broth (homemade or store-bought)
- 1/4 cup fresh basil leaves, chopped
- 1 teaspoon dried oregano
- 1 teaspoon dried thyme
- Salt and pepper, to taste

For Garnish:

- Fresh basil leaves
- Fresh thyme leaves
- Fresh oregano leaves

Instructions:

In a large pot, sauté onion, minced garlic, whole tomatoes, vegetable broth, dried oregano, and dried thyme until translucent. Add chopped fresh basil and let it simmer for 20-25 minutes. Use an immersion blender or regular blender to puree the soup until smooth and creamy. Season with salt and pepper to taste. Garnish with fresh basil leaves, thyme leaves, and oregano leaves. Enjoy this comforting and immune-boosting soup, which combines the richness of tomatoes and aromatic herbs for a delightful burst of flavor. Customize the soup with other herbs or spices, such as adding olive oil or Greek yogurt for added richness. Enjoy this immune-boosting soup.

8. Sweet Potato and Red Lentil Soup

Ingredients:

For the Soup:

- 2 tablespoons olive oil
- 1 onion, chopped
- 2 cloves garlic, minced
- 2 sweet potatoes, peeled and diced
- 1 cup red lentils, rinsed and drained
- 6 cups vegetable broth (homemade or store-bought)
- 1 teaspoon ground cumin
- 1 teaspoon ground coriander
- 1/2 teaspoon smoked paprika
- Salt and pepper, to taste

For Garnish:

- Fresh cilantro leaves, chopped
- Yogurt or coconut yogurt (optional)

Instructions:

In a large pot, sauté onion, minced garlic, diced sweet potatoes, rinsed red lentils, vegetable broth, ground cumin, ground coriander, and smoked paprika. Bring the mixture to a boil, reduce heat, cover, and simmer for 20-25 minutes until tender and red lentils are fully cooked. Puree the soup using an immersion blender or regular blender until smooth and creamy. Season with salt and pepper to taste. Garnish with fresh cilantro leaves and add yogurt or coconut yogurt if desired. Enjoy this hearty and immune-boosting soup, which combines the sweetness of sweet potatoes with the creaminess of red lentils. Customize the soup with other spices or herbs, such as adding chili flakes for a touch of heat.

C. Quinoa and Grain-Based Salads

1. Mediterranean Quinoa Salad

Ingredients:

For the Salad:

- 1 cup quinoa, rinsed and drained

- 2 cups water
- 1 cup cherry tomatoes, halved
- 1 cucumber, diced
- 1/2 cup Kalamata olives, pitted and sliced
- 1/2 cup red onion, finely chopped
- 1/2 cup crumbled feta cheese
- 1/4 cup fresh parsley, chopped

For the Dressing:

- 3 tablespoons extra-virgin olive oil
- 2 tablespoons lemon juice
- 2 cloves garlic, minced
- 1 teaspoon dried oregano
- Salt and black pepper to taste

Instructions:

In a medium saucepan, cook quinoa and water until cooked and absorbed. Cool. In a large salad bowl, combine quinoa, cherry tomatoes, cucumber, Kalamata olives, red onion, feta cheese, and fresh parsley. Create a dressing by whisking extra-virgin olive oil, lemon juice, minced garlic, dried oregano, salt, and black pepper. Pour the dressing over the salad and toss until well combined. Taste the salad and adjust seasoning if needed. Cover and refrigerate for at least 30 minutes before serving. Garnish with fresh parsley if desired.

2. *Greek-Inspired Farro Salad*

Ingredients:

For the Salad:

- 1 cup farro
- 2 cups water
- 1 cucumber, diced
- 1 cup cherry tomatoes, halved
- 1/2 red onion, finely chopped
- 1/2 cup Kalamata olives, pitted and sliced
- 1/2 cup crumbled feta cheese
- 1/4 cup fresh parsley, chopped

For the Dressing:

- 1/4 cup extra-virgin olive oil
- 3 tablespoons red wine vinegar
- 1 clove garlic, minced
- 1 teaspoon dried oregano
- Salt and black pepper to taste

Instructions:

To prepare a salad, boil farro and water in a medium saucepan, then simmer for 25-30 minutes until slightly chewy. Drain excess water and let it cool. In a large salad bowl, combine farro, cucumber, cherry tomatoes, red onion, Kalamata olives, feta cheese, and fresh parsley. In a separate bowl, whisk extra-virgin olive oil, red wine vinegar, minced garlic, dried oregano, salt, and black pepper to create a dressing. Pour the dressing over the salad and toss until well combined. Taste the salad and adjust seasoning if needed. Cover and refrigerate for at least 30 minutes before serving. Garnish with fresh parsley if desired.

3. Spicy Southwest Quinoa Salad

Ingredients:

For the Salad:
- 1 cup quinoa, rinsed and drained
- 2 cups water or vegetable broth
- 1 can (15 oz) black beans, drained and rinsed
- 1 cup corn kernels (fresh, frozen, or canned)
- 1 red bell pepper, diced
- 1/2 cup red onion, finely chopped
- 1/2 cup cherry tomatoes, halved
- 1/4 cup fresh cilantro, chopped
- 1/2 cup shredded cheddar cheese (optional)
- Avocado slices for garnish (optional)

For the Dressing:

- 1/4 cup extra-virgin olive oil
- 2 tablespoons lime juice
- 1 teaspoon ground cumin
- 1 teaspoon chili powder
- 1/2 teaspoon paprika
- 1/2 teaspoon cayenne pepper (adjust to your preferred level of spiciness)
- Salt and black pepper to taste

Instructions:

In a medium saucepan, boil the quinoa and vegetable broth together for 15 to 20 minutes, or until the quinoa is cooked. The cooked quinoa, black beans, corn, red bell pepper, red onion, cherry tomatoes, and fresh cilantro should all be combined in a big salad dish. Make the dressing in a separate bowl by combining the extra-virgin olive oil, lime juice, ground cumin, chili powder, paprika, cayenne pepper, salt, and black pepper. After pouring the dressing over the salad, mix to fully incorporate. If necessary, taste the salad and adjust the spice. Garnish with shredded cheddar cheese, if you'd like. Before serving, place the cover on and chill for a minimum of half an hour. If preferred, garnish with slices of avocado.

4. Citrus and Couscous Salad

Ingredients:

For the Salad:

- 1 cup couscous
- 1 1/4 cups water or vegetable broth
- 2 oranges, peeled and segmented
- 1 grapefruit, peeled and segmented
- 1/2 cup pomegranate seeds
- 1/4 cup chopped fresh mint leaves
- 1/4 cup sliced almonds, toasted
- 1/4 cup crumbled feta cheese (optional)

For the Dressing:

- 3 tablespoons extra-virgin olive oil
- 2 tablespoons fresh orange juice
- 2 tablespoons fresh grapefruit juice
- 1 tablespoon honey or maple syrup
- 1 teaspoon Dijon mustard
- Salt and black pepper to taste

Instructions:

In a medium saucepan, boil water or vegetable broth, stir in couscous, cover, and let sit for 5 minutes. Fluff with a fork and let it cool. In a large salad bowl, combine couscous, orange, grapefruit, pomegranate seeds, and mint leaves. In a separate bowl, whisk extra-virgin olive oil, juice, honey, mustard, salt, and black pepper to create a dressing. Pour dressing over salad and toss until well combined. Add toasted sliced almonds if desired and crumble feta cheese if using. Cover and refrigerate for at least 30 minutes before serving to allow flavors to meld.

5. *Tabbouleh with Bulgur Wheat*

Ingredients:

For the Salad:

- 1 cup fine bulgur wheat
- 2 cups boiling water
- 2 cups fresh parsley, finely chopped
- 1 cup fresh mint leaves, finely chopped
- 4 ripe tomatoes, diced
- 1/2 cup green onions, finely chopped
- 1/4 cup red onion, finely chopped
- 1/4 cup cucumber, finely chopped
- 1/4 cup extra-virgin olive oil
- 1/4 cup fresh lemon juice
- Salt and black pepper to taste

Instructions:

In order to make a tasty salad, place the fine bulgur wheat in a heatproof dish and boil it for 20 to 30 minutes, or until it becomes soft. Let it cool and fluff it up with a fork. The cooked and cooled bulgur, cucumber, tomatoes, green onions, red onions, parsley, and mint leaves should all be combined in a big salad dish. Mix the extra virgin olive oil and lemon juice in another bowl and add salt and black pepper to taste. After pouring the dressing over the salad, mix to fully incorporate. If necessary, taste the salad and adjust the spice. Before serving, place the cover on and chill for a minimum of half an hour. To ensure that all of the ingredients are well distributed, give the salad one last toss.

6. Wild Rice and Cranberry Salad

Ingredients:

For the Salad:

- 1 cup wild rice
- 3 cups water or vegetable broth
- 1/2 cup dried cranberries
- 1/2 cup chopped pecans or walnuts, toasted
- 1/4 cup chopped green onions
- 1/4 cup chopped fresh parsley
- 1/4 cup crumbled feta cheese (optional)

For the Dressing:

- 1/4 cup extra-virgin olive oil
- 2 tablespoons balsamic vinegar
- 1 tablespoon honey or maple syrup
- 1 teaspoon Dijon mustard
- Salt and black pepper to taste

Instructions:

In order to make this salad, you'll need wild rice, nuts or pecans, dried cranberries, green onions, and parsley. After the rice is cooked and allowed to cool, soak the cranberries in warm water. The dressing, which consists of extra-virgin olive oil, balsamic vinegar, honey, maple syrup, Dijon mustard, salt, and black pepper, is then mixed with the salad. After that, toss the salad with the dressing and, if desired, crumble the feta cheese. We taste the salad and add extra salt and pepper if necessary. To enable the flavors to mingle, cover and chill the salad for at least half an hour before serving.

7. Lentil and Brown Rice Salad

Ingredients:

For the Salad:

- 1 cup brown rice
- 1/2 cup green or brown lentils
- 2 1/2 cups water or vegetable broth
- 1/2 cup cucumber, diced
- 1/2 cup red bell pepper, diced
- 1/2 cup red onion, finely chopped
- 1/4 cup fresh parsley, chopped
- 1/4 cup feta cheese, crumbled (optional)

For the Dressing:

- 1/4 cup extra-virgin olive oil
- 3 tablespoons red wine vinegar
- 2 cloves garlic, minced
- 1 teaspoon Dijon mustard
- 1/2 teaspoon dried oregano
- Salt and black pepper to taste

Instructions:

Brown rice and lentils are cooked and soaked in broth in a saucepan. The rice is cooked and absorbed, while the lentils are rinsed and simmered for 20-25 minutes. Drain excess liquid and let them cool. In a large salad bowl, combine the cooked rice, lentils, cucumber, red bell pepper, onion, and parsley. In a separate bowl, whisk together extra-virgin olive oil, red wine vinegar, garlic, Dijon mustard, dried oregano, salt, and black pepper to create a dressing. Pour the dressing over the salad and toss it together. If using feta cheese, crumble it over the salad. Taste the salad and adjust the seasoning if needed. Cover and refrigerate for at least 30 minutes before serving to allow flavors to meld.

8. Israeli Couscous with Roasted Vegetables

Ingredients:

For the Israeli Couscous:

- 1 cup Israeli couscous (pearl couscous)
- 2 cups vegetable or chicken broth
- 1 tablespoon olive oil
- Salt and pepper, to taste

For the Roasted Vegetables:

- 2 cups mixed vegetables (e.g., bell peppers, zucchini, cherry tomatoes, red onion), cut into bite-sized pieces
- 2 tablespoons olive oil
- 1 teaspoon dried oregano
- Salt and pepper, to taste

For the Lemon-Herb Dressing:

- 2 tablespoons extra-virgin olive oil
- Juice of 1 lemon
- 2 tablespoons fresh basil, chopped
- 1 tablespoon fresh parsley, chopped
- Salt and pepper, to taste

Instructions:

For the Israeli Couscous

To make Israeli couscous, heat olive oil in a saucepan over medium heat and toast the couscous until browned. Add chicken or vegetable broth and season with pepper and salt, and heat until boiling. Reduce heat, cover, and simmer for 10-12 minutes. Fluff the couscous with a fork.

For the Roasted Vegetables

For the roasted vegetables, set the oven to 400°F or 200°C and toss mixed veggies, dried oregano, olive oil, salt, and pepper in a bowl. Arrange the vegetables in a single layer on a baking pan and roast for 20-25 minutes until soft and caramelized. Stir occasionally while roasting. Cool the vegetables before serving.

For the Lemon-Herb Dressing

For the dressing with lemon herb, combine extra-virgin olive oil, lemon juice, chopped fresh basil, parsley, salt, and pepper in a small dish. Place the roasted veggies and couscous in a large serving dish and drizzle with the lemon-herb dressing. Gently toss to mix.

This Israeli couscous with roasted vegetables is a delightful and fulfilling meal that blends the roasted sweetness of mixed vegetables, the brightness of the lemon-herb dressing, and the nutty taste of the couscous.

D. Anti-Inflammatory Broths and Stews

1. Turmeric and Ginger Lentil Stew

Ingredients:

For the Stew:

- 1 cup red or brown lentils, rinsed and drained
- 1 onion, finely chopped

- 2 carrots, peeled and diced
- 2 celery stalks, diced
- 2 cloves garlic, minced
- 1-inch piece of fresh ginger, peeled and grated
- 1 teaspoon ground turmeric
- 1 teaspoon ground cumin
- 1/2 teaspoon ground coriander
- 1/4 teaspoon red pepper flakes (adjust to your spice preference)
- 6 cups vegetable broth (homemade or store-bought)
- 1 can (14 ounces) diced tomatoes
- Salt and pepper, to taste
- Olive oil for sautéing

For Garnish:

- Fresh cilantro leaves, chopped
- Greek yogurt or coconut yogurt (optional)

Instructions:

In a large saucepan, heat olive oil and sauté diced carrots, celery, and onion for 5 minutes. Add grated ginger and garlic and cook for another minute or two. Add ground coriander, cumin, turmeric, and red pepper flakes and stir. Add washed lentils and stir. Add red lentils, canned diced tomatoes, and vegetable broth. Reduce heat, cover, and simmer for

25-30 minutes. Adjust seasoning to suit your taste. Ladle the Ginger and Turmeric Lentil Stew into bowls, top with fresh cilantro leaves, and, if desired, Greek or coconut yogurt. Enjoy the warming properties of turmeric and ginger, combined with the earthy goodness of lentils in this filling and immune-boosting stew.

2. Anti-Inflammatory Vegetable and Chickpea Soup

Ingredients:

For the Soup:

- 2 tablespoons olive oil
- 1 onion, finely chopped
- 2 carrots, peeled and diced
- 2 celery stalks, diced
- 2 cloves garlic, minced
- 1 teaspoon ground turmeric
- 1 teaspoon ground ginger
- 1 teaspoon ground cumin
- 1 can (15 ounces) chickpeas, drained and rinsed
- 4 cups vegetable broth (homemade or store-bought)
- 1 can (14 ounces) diced tomatoes
- 2 cups chopped spinach or kale
- Salt and pepper, to taste

For Garnish:

- Fresh cilantro or parsley, chopped
- Lemon wedges

Instructions:

In a large saucepan, sauté diced carrots, celery, and onion in olive oil over medium heat. Add minced garlic and sauté until fragrant. Add ground cumin, ginger, and turmeric, stirring to coat the veggies. Add chickpeas and stir into the spice blend. Add canned tomatoes and veggie broth, and simmer for 20-25 minutes. Add chopped kale or spinach and simmer for an additional two to three minutes. Adjust seasoning to suit your taste. Transfer the soup to individual bowls, top with parsley or cilantro, and serve with lemon slices. This nourishing and immune-stimulating soup blends anti-inflammatory spices, colorful veggies, and chickpeas. You can also add red pepper flakes or fresh lemon juice for extra flavor. Enjoy this nourishing and immune-stimulating soup.

3. Spicy Red Lentil and Kale Stew

Ingredients:

For the Stew:

- 1 cup red lentils, rinsed and drained
- 1 onion, finely chopped
- 2 cloves garlic, minced
- 1-inch piece of fresh ginger, peeled and grated
- 1 teaspoon ground cumin
- 1 teaspoon ground coriander
- 1/2 teaspoon cayenne pepper (adjust to your spice preference)
- 4 cups vegetable broth (homemade or store-bought)
- 1 can (14 ounces) diced tomatoes
- 4 cups fresh kale, stems removed and leaves chopped
- Salt and pepper, to taste
- Olive oil for sautéing

For Garnish:

- Fresh cilantro leaves, chopped
- Plain yogurt or coconut yogurt (optional)

Instructions:

In a large saucepan, heat olive oil and sauté onion, ginger, garlic, cayenne pepper, cumin, and coriander. Add red lentils and stir into the fragrant mixture. Add canned tomatoes and veggie broth, and simmer for 25 minutes. Add kale and cook for another two to three minutes. Season with salt and pepper to taste. Transfer the stew to bowls, top with plain or coconut yogurt, and decorate with fresh cilantro leaves. Enjoy the earthy taste of kale, the richness of red lentils, and the fire of spices in this delectable and immune-boosting Spicy Red Lentil and Kale Stew. Adjust seasoning to suit your taste. Enjoy the earthy goodness of kale, the richness of red lentils, and the fire of spices in this delectable and immune-boosting stew.

4. Tomato and Quinoa Detox Soup

Ingredients:

For the Soup:

- 1 cup quinoa, rinsed and drained
- 1 onion, finely chopped
- 2 cloves garlic, minced
- 2 carrots, peeled and diced
- 2 celery stalks, diced
- 1 can (28 ounces) crushed tomatoes
- 4 cups vegetable broth (homemade or store-bought)
- 1 teaspoon dried basil
- 1 teaspoon dried oregano
- Salt and pepper, to taste

- Olive oil for sautéing

For Garnish:

- Fresh basil leaves, chopped
- Grated Parmesan cheese (optional)

Instructions:

In a large saucepan, sauté diced carrots, celery, and onion in olive oil for 5 minutes. Add minced garlic and sauté until fragrant. Add dried oregano, basil, and rinsed quinoa, stirring to coat. Add vegetable broth and smashed tomatoes, and simmer for 20-25 minutes. Reduce heat and cover, and simmer quinoa for 20-25 minutes until soft. Adjust seasoning to suit taste. Transfer the soup to bowls, top with grated Parmesan cheese, and decorate with fresh basil leaves. Enjoy this immune-boosting Quinoa and Tomato Detox Soup, which combines the benefits of tomatoes with the nutrients of quinoa.

5. Miso and Seaweed Broth

Ingredients:

For the Broth:

- 4 cups water

- 4 cups vegetable broth (homemade or store-bought)
- 4-6 dried seaweed sheets (nori), torn into pieces
- 1/4 cup white miso paste
- 2 green onions (scallions), sliced
- 1 teaspoon sesame oil
- 1 teaspoon soy sauce (optional)
- Salt and pepper, to taste

For Garnish:

- Toasted sesame seeds
- Thinly sliced fresh ginger

Instructions:

In a large saucepan, heat 4 cups water and 4 cups vegetable broth to a mild boil. Add dried seaweed sheets and simmer for 5 to 7 minutes until soft and flavorful. Dilute miso paste in a small dish to make it easier to integrate into the soup. Mix broth with diluted miso paste, avoiding boiling to maintain taste. Fill the broth with cut green onions and season with soy sauce and sesame oil. Adjust seasoning with salt and pepper. Turn off heat and serve in individual bowls with thinly sliced fresh ginger and toasted sesame seeds. Enjoy the umami of miso and marine tastes of seaweed in this calming and immune-boosting soup.

6. Roasted Butternut Squash Soup with Turmeric

Ingredients:

For the Soup:

- 1 medium butternut squash, peeled, seeded, and cubed
- 1 onion, chopped
- 2 cloves garlic, minced
- 2 carrots, peeled and diced
- 2 apples, peeled, cored, and diced
- 4 cups vegetable broth (homemade or store-bought)
- 1 can (14 ounces) coconut milk
- 1 teaspoon ground turmeric
- 1/2 teaspoon ground cinnamon
- Olive oil for roasting
- Salt and pepper, to taste

For Garnish:

- Fresh cilantro leaves, chopped
- Drizzle of coconut milk (optional)

Instructions:

For Roasting the Butternut Squash:

Preheat the oven to 400°F or 200°C. Mix olive oil, salt, and pepper with cubed butternut squash. Arrange the squash in a single layer on a baking pan. Roast for 30 to 35 minutes until soft and caramelized, stirring occasionally.

For the Soup:

In a large saucepan, sauté onion, garlic, apples, carrots, and butternut squash in olive oil for three to four minutes. Add ground cinnamon, turmeric, and vegetable broth, and simmer for five minutes. Lower heat, cover, and simmer for 15 to 20 minutes to combine flavors. Puree the soup using an immersion blender or standard blender until creamy and smooth. Add coconut milk for a tropical taste. Season with salt and pepper to taste. Spoon the soup into bowls, top with fresh cilantro leaves, and drizzle with coconut milk if desired. Enjoy this soothing and immune-boosting soup, which blends the warmth of turmeric, the smoothness of coconut milk, and the sweetness of butternut squash.

7. Lemon and Herb Chicken Broth

Ingredients:

For the Broth:

- 4 cups chicken broth (homemade or store-bought)
- 2 boneless, skinless chicken breasts
- 1 lemon, sliced
- 4 sprigs fresh rosemary
- 4 sprigs fresh thyme
- 2 bay leaves
- Salt and pepper, to taste

For Garnish:

- Fresh parsley leaves, chopped
- Lemon wedges

Instructions:

In a large saucepan, boil chicken broth over medium heat. Add skinless, boneless chicken breasts, lemon slices, bay leaves, fresh thyme and rosemary, salt, and pepper. Simmer for 20-25 minutes until cooked and soft. Shred the chicken into bite-sized pieces and add back to the broth. Discard herb sprigs and bay leaves. Add more salt and pepper if needed. Serve the Lemon and Herb Chicken Broth in dishes, top with lemon wedges and fresh parsley leaves. Enjoy the comforting aromas of chicken and herbs in this immune-boosting and calming broth.

8. Cauliflower and Turmeric Coconut Soup

Ingredients:

For the Soup:

- 1 head of cauliflower, cut into florets
- 1 onion, chopped
- 2 cloves garlic, minced
- 1 can (14 ounces) coconut milk
- 4 cups vegetable broth (homemade or store-bought)
- 1 teaspoon ground turmeric
- 1/2 teaspoon ground cumin
- 1/2 teaspoon ground coriander
- Olive oil for sautéing
- Salt and pepper, to taste

For Garnish:

- Fresh cilantro leaves, chopped
- Toasted coconut flakes

Instructions:

In a large saucepan, sauté onion, minced garlic, and cauliflower florets over medium heat. Add ground coriander, cumin, and turmeric to the pan and cook until fragrant. Add vegetable broth and simmer for 20-25 minutes until soft. Puree the soup using an immersion blender or standard blender until creamy and smooth. Add a can of coconut milk for a tropical taste. Season with salt and pepper to taste. Spoon the soup into bowls and garnish with toasted coconut flakes and fresh cilantro leaves. Enjoy the richness of coconut, turmeric, and cauliflower in this immune-boosting soup. Adjust seasoning to suit your taste. Enjoy the richness of coconut, turmeric, and cauliflower in this velvety, immune-boosting soup.

CHAPTER 3: NUTRIENT-RICH MAIN COURSES

A. Lean Protein Powerhouses

1. Grilled Lemon Herb Chicken

Ingredients:

- 1/4 cup olive oil
- 2 lemons, juiced and zested
- 3 cloves garlic, minced
- 2 tablespoons fresh rosemary, chopped
- 2 tablespoons fresh thyme, chopped
- Salt and black pepper, to taste
- 4 boneless, skinless chicken breasts
- Additional lemon slices for grilling (optional)
- Fresh herbs for garnish (rosemary and thyme sprigs)

Instructions:

In a small bowl, combine olive oil, lemon zest, lemon juice, minced garlic, rosemary, and thyme. Add salt and black pepper to taste. Place chicken breasts in a plastic bag or shallow plate and cover with the Lemon Herb Marinade. Marinate for at least 30 minutes or up to 4 hours for a stronger taste. Set the grill to medium-high and oil the grill grates. Remove the chicken from the marinade and grill for 6-8 minutes on each side, or until no longer pink in the middle and internal temperature reaches 165°F (74°C). If desired, cook lemon slices for a few minutes on each side. Remove the chicken from the grill and allow it to rest. Cut the Grilled Lemon Herb Chicken into slices and sprinkle with fresh herbs like thyme and rosemary sprigs. Serve the chicken with the grilled lemon segments. Enjoy this tasty and healthy Grilled Lemon Herb Chicken with a revitalizing blend of herbs and citrus.

2. Seared Tofu with Peanut Sauce

Ingredients:

For the Tofu:

- 1 block extra-firm tofu, pressed and cut into cubes
- 2 tablespoons soy sauce or tamari
- 1 tablespoon sesame oil

- 1 teaspoon ground ginger
- 1 teaspoon garlic powder
- Salt and pepper, to taste
- Cooking oil for searing

For the Peanut Sauce:

- 1/4 cup natural peanut butter
- 2 tablespoons soy sauce or tamari
- 1 tablespoon rice vinegar
- 1 tablespoon honey or maple syrup
- 1 teaspoon sesame oil
- 1 teaspoon sriracha sauce (adjust to your spice preference)
- 2-3 tablespoons water (for desired consistency)

For Garnish:

- Chopped green onions
- Crushed peanuts
- Sesame seeds

Instructions:

To prepare the tofu, press it to remove excess liquid, cut it into bite-sized pieces, and marinate it in a mixture of sesame oil, ground ginger, garlic powder, soy sauce, salt, and pepper. Allow the tofu to rest for ten to fifteen minutes to absorb the flavors.

Sear the tofu in a pan over medium-high heat, ensuring it is not packed too tightly. Sear for 2-3 minutes on each side until brown and slightly crispy. Remove the tofu and set it aside.

To prepare the peanut sauce, combine natural peanut butter, tamari or soy sauce, rice vinegar, honey, sesame oil, and sriracha sauce in a small bowl. Gradually add water to achieve the desired consistency and whisk until smooth. Pour the peanut sauce over the seared tofu, add sesame seeds, crushed peanuts, and sliced green onions as a garnish. Enjoy this flavorful and high-protein seared tofu with peanut sauce as a main course or with noodles or rice of your choice.

3. Baked Salmon with Dill and Asparagus

Ingredients:

For the Salmon:

- 4 salmon filets
- 2 tablespoons olive oil
- 2 cloves garlic, minced
- 1 lemon, thinly sliced
- Salt and black pepper, to taste
- Fresh dill sprigs for garnish

For the Asparagus:

- 1 bunch of asparagus, woody ends trimmed
- 1 tablespoon olive oil
- Salt and black pepper, to taste

For the Lemon-Dill Sauce:

- 1/4 cup mayonnaise
- 2 tablespoons fresh dill, finely chopped
- 1 tablespoon lemon juice
- 1 teaspoon lemon zest
- Salt and black pepper, to taste

Instructions:

To prepare the salmon, set the oven to 375°F or 190°C, arrange the salmon filets on a baking pan, season with salt, black pepper, and garlic, and drizzle with olive oil. Place lemon wedges over the salmon and bake for 12 to 15 minutes until cooked to your preferred doneness. Meanwhile, toss the trimmed asparagus with olive oil, salt, and black pepper while the salmon is baking. Roast the asparagus on a separate baking sheet for the last ten minutes of the salmon's cooking. In a small bowl, combine mayonnaise, lemon juice, zest, chopped fresh dill, salt, and black pepper, taste and adjust the sauce's flavor. Transfer the cooked salmon filets to a plate, arrange the salmon and asparagus in a circle, cover with the lemon-dill sauce, and add fresh dill sprigs for visual appeal. Enjoy this delicious Baked Salmon with Dill and Asparagus for a balanced dinner.

4. Quinoa and Black Bean Stuffed Peppers

Ingredients:

For the Stuffed Peppers:

- 4 large bell peppers, any color
- 1 cup quinoa, rinsed and drained
- 2 cups vegetable broth (homemade or store-bought)
- 1 can (15 ounces) black beans, drained and rinsed
- 1 cup corn kernels (fresh, frozen, or canned)
- 1 cup diced tomatoes (canned or fresh)
- 1 teaspoon ground cumin
- 1 teaspoon chili powder
- 1/2 teaspoon garlic powder
- Salt and pepper, to taste
- 1 cup shredded cheddar or vegan cheese (optional)

For Garnish:

- Fresh cilantro, chopped

- Sour cream or vegan yogurt (optional)

Instructions:

To prepare the Quinoa and Black Bean Stuffed Peppers, bring vegetable broth to a boil, then stir in the quinoa and cook for 15-20 minutes. Fluff the quinoa and set aside. Preheat the oven to 375°F or 190°C. Cut off the bell peppers' tops to extract seeds and membranes. In a large bowl, mix the cooked quinoa, diced tomatoes, black beans, corn, ground cumin, chili powder, garlic powder, salt, and pepper. Stuff each pepper with the mixture and transfer them to an aluminum foil-covered baking tray. Bake for 25-30 minutes or until soft. If desired, cover the peppers with shredded cheese and bake for an additional five to ten minutes. Remove the foil, cover the peppers with cheese, and bake for an additional five to ten minutes. Once cooled, garnish with fresh cilantro and serve with vegan yogurt or sour cream. Enjoy the savory and visually stunning Quinoa and Black Bean Stuffed Peppers, a filling and healthy meal.

5. Greek Yogurt and Berry Parfait

Ingredients:

- 2 cups Greek yogurt (plain or vanilla flavored)

- 1 cup mixed berries (strawberries, blueberries, raspberries, blackberries)
- 1/2 cup granola
- 2 tablespoons honey or maple syrup (optional)
- Fresh mint leaves for garnish (optional)

Instructions:

To create a Greek Yogurt and Berry Parfait, start by adding 1/4 cup of yogurt to the bottom of a glass or parfait dish. Layer 1/4 cup of mixed berries, drizzle with granola, and repeat with more yogurt, granola, and mixed berries. Add honey or maple syrup for sweetness. Garnish with mint leaves for color. Repeat with remaining ingredients. Serve immediately or chill for a refreshing treat. Enjoy this nutritious and tasty treat for breakfast, snack, or dessert.

6. Spicy Grilled Shrimp Skewers

Ingredients:

For the Shrimp:

- 1 pound large shrimp, peeled and deveined
- 2 tablespoons olive oil
- 2 cloves garlic, minced
- 1 teaspoon paprika

- 1/2 teaspoon cayenne pepper (adjust to your spice preference)
- Salt and black pepper, to taste
- Wooden skewers, soaked in water

For Garnish:

- Fresh cilantro leaves, chopped
- Lemon wedges

Instructions:

To prepare shrimp, combine olive oil, paprika, cayenne pepper, garlic, salt, and black pepper in a bowl. Place peeled and deveined shrimp in the bowl and coat them in the marinade for 15-30 minutes. Turn the heat up to medium-high on the grill and secure the marinated shrimp onto wooden skewers. Grill for two to three minutes each side until they turn pink and become slightly scorched. Remove the skewers, serve with lemon slices and fresh cilantro leaves. Adjust the heat of cayenne pepper to suit your taste. Enjoy these delicious grilled shrimp skewers as a main course or appetizer.

7. Lentil and Vegetable Stir-Fry

Ingredients:

For the Stir-Fry:

- 1 cup brown or green lentils, cooked and drained
- 2 cups mixed vegetables (e.g., bell peppers, broccoli, carrots, snap peas)
- 1 tablespoon vegetable oil
- 2 cloves garlic, minced
- 1-inch piece of ginger, minced
- 1 tablespoon soy sauce or tamari
- 1 tablespoon hoisin sauce
- Salt and black pepper, to taste

For Garnish:

- Fresh cilantro leaves, chopped
- Sesame seeds

Instructions:

To prepare lentils, follow the packet's instructions and drain them. Heat vegetable oil in a large skillet or wok and stir-fry ginger and minced garlic for a minute. Add mixed vegetables and stir-fry for five to seven minutes until crisp-tender and slightly browned. Add hoisin sauce, black pepper, salt, and soy sauce or tamari, discarding to coat. Toss in cooked lentils and stir-fry for two to three minutes.

Receive the stir-fried vegetables and lentils, spoon them into bowls or serving plates, sprinkle fresh cilantro leaves and sesame seeds for a visual and taste boost. Enjoy this filling and healthy plant-based dinner, and feel free to adjust the vegetable choices to suit your taste.

B. Colorful Vegetable Stir-Fries

1. Rainbow Bell Pepper Stir-Fry

Ingredients:

For the Stir-Fry:

- 2 red bell peppers, thinly sliced
- 2 yellow bell peppers, thinly sliced
- 2 green bell peppers, thinly sliced
- 2 orange bell peppers, thinly sliced
- 1 red onion, thinly sliced
- 2 cloves garlic, minced
- 1 tablespoon vegetable oil
- 1 teaspoon sesame oil (optional)
- Salt and black pepper, to taste

For the Stir-Fry Sauce:

- 1/4 cup soy sauce or tamari
- 2 tablespoons rice vinegar
- 1 tablespoon honey or maple syrup
- 1 teaspoon fresh ginger, grated
- 1 teaspoon cornstarch (to thicken the sauce)
- Sesame seeds for garnish (optional)
- Fresh cilantro leaves for garnish (optional)

Instructions:

To make a Rainbow Bell Pepper Stir-Fry, combine rice vinegar, grated ginger, honey, maple syrup, soy sauce or tamari, and cornstarch in a small basin. Heat vegetable oil over high heat, add minced garlic, red onion, and cut bell peppers, stir-fry for five to seven minutes until crisp-tender and charred. Drizzle the vegetables with the stir-fry sauce and let it thicken for two to three minutes. For extra flavor, sprinkle sesame oil over the stir-fry. Serve the Rainbow Bell Pepper Stir-Fry on a dish, garnish with sesame seeds and fresh cilantro leaves. This healthy and delicious dish can be served as a main meal or a colorful side dish, and can be made a full dinner by adding protein sources like shrimp, chicken, or tofu.

2. Broccoli and Snap Pea Stir-Fry

Ingredients:

For the Stir-Fry:

- 2 cups broccoli florets
- 2 cups snap peas, ends trimmed
- 1 red bell pepper, thinly sliced
- 1 yellow bell pepper, thinly sliced
- 1 small red onion, thinly sliced
- 2 cloves garlic, minced
- 1 tablespoon vegetable oil
- 1 tablespoon sesame oil (optional)
- Salt and black pepper, to taste

For the Stir-Fry Sauce:

- 1/4 cup soy sauce or tamari
- 2 tablespoons rice vinegar
- 1 tablespoon honey or maple syrup
- 1 teaspoon fresh ginger, grated
- 1 teaspoon cornstarch (to thicken the sauce)
- Sesame seeds for garnish (optional)
- Sliced green onions for garnish (optional)

Instructions:

To make a stir-fried broccoli and snap peas dish, combine rice vinegar, grated ginger, honey, maple syrup, soy sauce, and cornstarch in a small basin. Heat vegetable oil over high heat and add minced garlic. Stir-fry broccoli florets, snap peas, red onion, yellow bell pepper, and red bell pepper for five to seven minutes until crisp-tender and charred. Drizzle the vegetables with the stir-fry sauce and let it thicken for two to three minutes. For extra flavor, sprinkle sesame oil over the stir-fry. Serve the stir-fried broccoli and snap peas on a serving plate, garnish with green onions and sesame seeds. This dish can be served as a filling and healthy side dish or main entrée, and can be topped with protein sources like shrimp, chicken, or tofu.

3. Sweet and Sour Pineapple Stir-Fry

Ingredients:

For the Stir-Fry:

- 1 cup pineapple chunks (fresh or canned)
- 1 red bell pepper, cut into chunks
- 1 green bell pepper, cut into chunks
- 1 small red onion, thinly sliced
- 1 cup snow peas
- 1 cup broccoli florets
- 1 cup carrots, sliced into thin rounds
- 2 cloves garlic, minced
- 2 tablespoons vegetable oil

- Salt and black pepper, to taste

For the Sweet and Sour Sauce:

- 1/2 cup pineapple juice (from the canned pineapple, if using)
- 3 tablespoons rice vinegar
- 2 tablespoons ketchup
- 2 tablespoons honey or brown sugar
- 1 tablespoon soy sauce or tamari
- 1 tablespoon cornstarch
- 1/2 teaspoon fresh ginger, grated
- Sesame seeds and chopped green onions for garnish (optional)

Instructions:

In this recipe, pineapple juice, ketchup, rice vinegar, honey, brown sugar, soy sauce, tamari, cornstarch, and grated ginger are mixed in a bowl. The vegetables are sautéd in vegetable oil over medium-high heat, with minced garlic and broccoli, carrots, snow peas, red onion, green bell pepper, and red bell pepper. The vegetables are stir-fried for five to seven minutes until crisp-tender and have a hint of char. The sweet and sour sauce is then added to the vegetables and pineapple pieces, allowing the sauce to thicken. The dish is served on a serving plate, garnished with chopped green onions and sesame seeds for extra flavor. For a full supper, it can be served with noodles or steaming rice.

4. Spicy Thai Basil Vegetable Stir-Fry

Ingredients:

For the Stir-Fry:

- 2 cups mixed vegetables (e.g., bell peppers, broccoli, carrots, snap peas)
- 1 tablespoon vegetable oil
- 2 cloves garlic, minced
- 1 red chili pepper, thinly sliced (adjust to your spice preference)
- 1 cup tofu, cubed (optional)
- Fresh basil leaves, torn

For the Stir-Fry Sauce:

- 2 tablespoons soy sauce or tamari
- 1 tablespoon oyster sauce or vegetarian oyster sauce (for a vegetarian option)
- 1 teaspoon fish sauce or soy sauce (for a vegetarian option)
- 1 teaspoon brown sugar
- 1/2 teaspoon fresh ginger, grated

Instructions:

To make Thai basil vegetable stir-fried, combine soy sauce, brown sugar, grated ginger, oyster sauce, fish sauce, and oyster sauce in a small dish. Heat vegetable oil in a large skillet or wok over medium-high heat and sauté red chili pepper slices and chopped garlic until aromatic. Add cubed tofu and stir-fry for three to four minutes, or until soft and crisp. Add tofu and veggies and stir-fry for 5 to 7 minutes. Drizzle the stir-fried sauce over the vegetables and toss to coat. Simmer for two to three minutes. Place the stir-fry on a serving plate and scatter fresh basil leaves over it for an enhanced taste and appearance. Adjust the spice level to suit your preferred heat. Serve with noodles or steamed rice for a full dinner.

5. *Teriyaki Bok Choy and Mushroom Stir-Fry*

Ingredients:

For the Stir-Fry:

- 2 baby bok choy heads, sliced into bite-sized pieces
- 8 ounces mushrooms (shiitake, cremini, or your choice), sliced
- 2 cloves garlic, minced
- 1 tablespoon vegetable oil

- 1 cup cooked brown rice or noodles

For the Teriyaki Sauce:

- 1/4 cup soy sauce or tamari
- 2 tablespoons honey or brown sugar
- 1 tablespoon rice vinegar
- 1 teaspoon fresh ginger, grated
- 1/2 teaspoon cornstarch

For Garnish:

- Toasted sesame seeds
- Sliced green onions

Instructions:

To make Teriyaki Sauce, combine rice vinegar, grated ginger, honey, brown sugar, soy sauce, and cornstarch in a small basin. Heat vegetable oil over medium-high heat and sauté minced garlic for 30 seconds. Add bok choy and sliced mushrooms, stir-fried for five to seven minutes. Drizzle the sauce over the vegetables, stirring to ensure a uniform coating. Simmer for two to three minutes until thickened. Serve the Teriyaki Bok Choy and Mushroom Stir-Fry over brown rice or noodles, garnish with green onions and toasted sesame seeds. This flavorful and filling stir-fry can be served as a tasty and nourishing supper, or with tofu, chicken, shrimp, or other protein for a satisfying dinner.

6. Sesame Ginger Zucchini Stir-Fry

Ingredients:

For the Stir-Fry:

- 4 medium zucchini, cut into thin strips or rounds
- 2 tablespoons vegetable oil
- 2 cloves garlic, minced
- 1 tablespoon fresh ginger, grated
- 1 red bell pepper, thinly sliced
- 1 yellow bell pepper, thinly sliced
- 1 cup snow peas, ends trimmed
- 1 cup baby corn, halved
- 1/4 cup sesame seeds

For the Stir-Fry Sauce:

- 1/4 cup soy sauce or tamari
- 2 tablespoons rice vinegar
- 1 tablespoon honey or brown sugar
- 1 teaspoon sesame oil
- 1/2 teaspoon cornstarch

Instructions:

To prepare the Sesame Ginger Zucchini Stir-Fry, whisk together soy sauce, rice vinegar, honey, sesame oil, and cornstarch. Heat vegetable oil in a large skillet over medium-high heat and sauté minced garlic and grated ginger for 30 seconds. Add sliced zucchini, red bell pepper, yellow bell pepper, snow peas, and baby corn and stir-fry for 5-7 minutes until tender-crisp and slightly charred. Pour the stir-fry sauce over the vegetables and toss to coat evenly. Cook for an additional 2-3 minutes until the sauce thickens. Serve the stir-fry on a serving platter and sprinkle sesame seeds for added flavor. Enjoy this nutritious main course with steamed rice or noodles or add your preferred protein source like tofu, chicken, or shrimp.

7. Eggplant and Red Pepper Stir-Fry

Ingredients:

For the Stir-Fry:

- 1 large eggplant, cut into bite-sized pieces
- 2 red bell peppers, thinly sliced
- 1 onion, thinly sliced
- 2 cloves garlic, minced
- 2 tablespoons vegetable oil
- Salt and black pepper, to taste

For the Stir-Fry Sauce:

- 1/4 cup soy sauce or tamari
- 2 tablespoons rice vinegar
- 1 tablespoon honey or brown sugar
- 1 teaspoon fresh ginger, grated
- 1/2 teaspoon cornstarch

Instructions:

To make a stir-fried eggplant and red pepper dish, combine rice vinegar, soy sauce, ginger, honey, and cornstarch in a small dish. Heat vegetable oil in a large skillet and sauté minced garlic for 30 seconds. Add onion, bell peppers, and eggplant and stir-fry for ten to twelve minutes. Season with salt and black pepper to taste. Drizzle the vegetables with the stir-fry sauce and simmer for two to three minutes. Serve the dish with fresh cilantro leaves for visual appeal and taste. For a full dinner, serve it with noodles or steaming rice, and add your favorite protein source like shrimp, chicken, or tofu.

D. Mediterranean and Plant-Based Delights

1. Greek Chickpea Salad

Ingredients:

For the Salad:

- 2 cans (15 ounces each) chickpeas, drained and rinsed
- 1 cucumber, diced
- 1 cup cherry tomatoes, halved
- 1 red onion, finely chopped
- 1/2 cup Kalamata olives, pitted and sliced
- 1/2 cup crumbled feta cheese
- 1/4 cup fresh parsley, chopped
- 1/4 cup fresh mint, chopped

For the Dressing:

- 1/4 cup extra-virgin olive oil
- 3 tablespoons red wine vinegar
- 1 teaspoon dried oregano
- Salt and black pepper, to taste

Instructions:

To prepare the Greek Chickpea Salad, combine extra virgin olive oil, red wine vinegar, black pepper, salt, and dried oregano in a small dish. In a large bowl, combine chopped red onion, diced cucumber, feta cheese, cherry tomatoes, sliced Kalamata olives, and chickpeas. Top with fresh parsley and mint. Drizzle the salad with the dressing and gently mix. Serve immediately or refrigerate for flavor mingling. Enjoy this nutritious and filling salad as an accompaniment to a main course or as a standalone meal.

2. Mediterranean Roasted Vegetable Platter

Ingredients:

For the Roasted Vegetables:

- 2 large red bell peppers, cut into strips
- 2 zucchinis, sliced into rounds
- 1 large eggplant, sliced into rounds
- 1 red onion, cut into wedges
- 1 pint cherry tomatoes
- 2 tablespoons extra-virgin olive oil
- Salt and black pepper, to taste
- 2 cloves garlic, minced
- 1 teaspoon dried oregano
- 1 teaspoon dried thyme
- 1 teaspoon dried rosemary (or fresh sprigs)

- 1 lemon, sliced into rounds (for garnish)
- Fresh parsley, chopped (for garnish)

For the Yogurt Sauce:

- 1 cup Greek yogurt
- 2 tablespoons extra-virgin olive oil
- 1 lemon, juiced
- 2 cloves garlic, minced
- 1 teaspoon dried dill (or fresh dill)
- Salt and black pepper, to taste

Instructions:

Preheat your oven to 425°F (220°C). In a large mixing bowl, combine red bell peppers, zucchini, eggplant, red onion, cherry tomatoes, and lemon slices. Drizzle extra-virgin olive oil over the vegetables and season with minced garlic, dried oregano, dried thyme, dried rosemary, salt, and black pepper. Arrange the vegetables in a single layer on a baking sheet and roast for 25-30 minutes until tender and slightly caramelized. In a separate bowl, mix Greek yogurt, extra-virgin olive oil, lemon juice, minced garlic, dried dill, salt, and black pepper. Transfer the roasted vegetables to a serving platter, drizzle the yogurt sauce over the vegetables or serve it on the side. Garnish with fresh parsley. Serve this Mediterranean Roasted

Vegetable Platter as a colorful side dish or appetizer, or pair it with pita bread, hummus, or grilled meat or fish.

3. Falafel with Tahini Sauce

Ingredients:

For the Falafel:

- 2 cups canned chickpeas, drained and rinsed
- 1/2 large onion, roughly chopped
- 2-3 cloves garlic, minced
- 1/4 cup fresh parsley, chopped
- 1/4 cup fresh cilantro, chopped
- 1 teaspoon cumin
- 1 teaspoon coriander
- 1/4 teaspoon cayenne pepper (adjust to your spice preference)
- Salt and black pepper, to taste
- 1 teaspoon baking powder
- 3-4 tablespoons all-purpose flour
- Vegetable oil for frying

For the Tahini Sauce:

- 1/2 cup tahini
- 2 cloves garlic, minced
- 1/4 cup fresh lemon juice

- 2 tablespoons water
- 2 tablespoons extra-virgin olive oil
- Salt, to taste

For Serving:

- Pita bread or flatbreads
- Sliced tomatoes
- Sliced cucumbers
- Fresh lettuce or greens
- Sliced red onion

Instructions:

To make falafel, blend chickpeas, onion, garlic, cilantro, parsley, cumin, coriander, cayenne pepper, salt, and black pepper in a food processor. Add all-purpose flour and baking powder to the falafel mixture, making it stiff enough to hold together. Form the mixture into small patties and fry them in vegetable oil for 3-4 minutes on each side until crispy and golden brown. Drain on paper towels. To prepare the tahini sauce, combine tahini, water, extra-virgin olive oil, minced garlic, lemon juice, and salt in a small bowl. If necessary, add more water to thin the consistency. Top the falafel with sliced tomatoes, cucumbers, red onion, and lettuce, and serve on flatbreads or pita bread. Cover the falafel and vegetables with tahini sauce, and enjoy this delectable falafel as a filling or tasty wrap or sandwich.

4. Caprese Stuffed Portobello Mushrooms

Ingredients:

For the Stuffed Mushrooms:

- 4 large Portobello mushrooms, stems removed and cleaned
- 2 tablespoons extra-virgin olive oil
- 2 cloves garlic, minced
- Salt and black pepper, to taste
- 1 1/2 cups fresh mozzarella cheese, shredded or sliced
- 1 cup cherry tomatoes, halved
- 1/4 cup fresh basil leaves, chopped
- Balsamic glaze (for drizzling, optional)

For the Pesto Drizzle (optional):

- 1/2 cup fresh basil leaves
- 1/4 cup grated Parmesan cheese
- 1/4 cup pine nuts
- 2 cloves garlic
- 1/4 cup extra-virgin olive oil
- Salt and black pepper, to taste

Instructions:

Turn the oven on to 375°F, or 190°C. Add a little extra virgin olive oil to the Portobello mushrooms and season with salt, black pepper, and garlic. Put the gill side up on a baking sheet and stuff a piece of mozzarella cheese into each mushroom. Add cherry tomato halves on top. Bake the mushrooms for 15 to 20 minutes, or until the cheese is melted and soft. Take out of the oven and top with freshly chopped basil leaves. Drizzle the mushrooms with balsamic glaze, if preferred. In order to make the Pesto Drizzle, place the garlic, pine nuts, basil leaves, extra virgin olive oil, salt, and black pepper in a food processor. Before serving, drizzle the pesto over the mushrooms. Savor the bright tastes of Caprese as an appetizer or a light main dish.

5. Ratatouille with Herbed Quinoa

Ingredients:

For the Ratatouille:

- 2 tablespoons olive oil
- 1 onion, chopped
- 3 cloves garlic, minced
- 1 eggplant, diced
- 2 zucchinis, diced

- 1 red bell pepper, diced
- 1 yellow bell pepper, diced
- 1 can (14 ounces) crushed tomatoes
- 1 can (14 ounces) diced tomatoes
- 1 teaspoon dried thyme
- 1 teaspoon dried oregano
- Salt and black pepper, to taste
- Fresh basil leaves, for garnish

For the Herbed Quinoa:

- 1 cup quinoa, rinsed and drained
- 2 cups vegetable broth or water
- 1 teaspoon dried basil
- 1 teaspoon dried parsley
- Salt and black pepper, to taste

Instructions:

To make Ratatouille, heat olive oil in a large pot over medium heat. Add onion, garlic, eggplant, zucchinis, red and yellow bell peppers, crushed tomatoes, and season with dried thyme, oregano, salt, and black pepper. Sauté for 8-10 minutes until vegetables soften. Add crushed tomatoes and diced tomatoes, season with dried thyme, oregano, salt, and black pepper. Reduce heat, cover, and simmer for 20-25 minutes until vegetables are tender and flavors meld. Adjust seasoning as needed.

For Herbed Quinoa, combine quinoa, vegetable broth, basil, parsley, salt, and black pepper in a separate saucepan. Bring to a boil, then reduce heat to low, cover, and simmer for 15-20 minutes until quinoa is cooked and liquid is absorbed. Serve the Ratatouille over Herbed Quinoa and garnish with fresh basil leaves for added flavor. Enjoy this wholesome and nutritious main course.

6. Greek Lentil and Spinach Stew

Ingredients:

- 1 cup green or brown lentils, rinsed and drained
- 2 tablespoons olive oil
- 1 onion, finely chopped
- 3 cloves garlic, minced
- 1 carrot, diced
- 1 celery stalk, diced
- 1 red bell pepper, diced
- 1 can (14 ounces) diced tomatoes
- 1 teaspoon dried oregano
- 1 teaspoon dried thyme
- 4 cups vegetable broth
- 4 cups fresh spinach, chopped
- Salt and black pepper, to taste
- Crumbled feta cheese for garnish (optional)
- Fresh lemon wedges for serving

Instructions:

In a large saucepan, heat olive oil over medium heat and sauté onion, garlic, red bell pepper, celery, and carrot for three to four minutes. Add dried thyme, oregano, and tomatoes, and mix well. Fill the saucepan with washed lentils and vegetable broth, season with salt and black pepper, and boil until soft. Reduce heat, cover, and simmer for 25 to 30 minutes. Add chopped fresh spinach and allow it to wilt. Taste and adjust seasoning as needed. Serve the Spinach and Lentil Stew in dishes, garnish with crumbled feta cheese, and serve with fresh lemon wedges. This filling and nourishing Greek Lentil and Spinach Stew is a substantial and nourishing dinner option.

7. Mediterranean Couscous with Roasted Red Pepper Pesto

Ingredients:

For the Couscous:

- 1 cup couscous
- 1 1/4 cups vegetable broth or water
- 1 tablespoon olive oil
- 1/2 cup sun-dried tomatoes, chopped

- 1/4 cup Kalamata olives, pitted and chopped
- 1/4 cup crumbled feta cheese
- 2 tablespoons fresh parsley, chopped
- Salt and black pepper, to taste

For the Roasted Red Pepper Pesto:

- 2 large red bell peppers, roasted, peeled, and seeded
- 1/4 cup pine nuts
- 2 cloves garlic, minced
- 1/4 cup grated Parmesan cheese
- 1/4 cup extra-virgin olive oil
- Salt and black pepper, to taste

Instructions:

This recipe involves roasting red bell peppers on a grill or in the oven until charred. After cooling, chop the roasted peppers and process them in a food processor with pine nuts, minced garlic, grated Parmesan cheese, and extra-virgin olive oil. Season with salt and black pepper to taste.

For the Mediterranean Couscous, boil vegetable broth or water, stir in couscous and olive oil, and let it sit for 5 minutes. Fluff the couscous with a fork, then add sun-dried tomatoes, Kalamata olives, crumbled feta cheese, and chopped fresh parsley. Toss to combine.

Serve the Mediterranean Couscous with Roasted Red Pepper Pesto over the couscous, serving it as a flavorful side dish or a light main course. Enjoy this vibrant Mediterranean Couscous as a flavorful and vibrant side dish or a light main course.

E. Seafood Specials for Radiant Skin

1. Baked Salmon with Lemon-Dill Sauce

Ingredients:

For the Baked Salmon:

- 4 salmon filets
- 2 tablespoons olive oil
- 2 cloves garlic, minced
- 1 lemon, sliced
- Salt and black pepper, to taste
- Fresh dill sprigs, for garnish

For the Lemon-Dill Sauce:

- 1/2 cup Greek yogurt
- 1 lemon, juiced
- 2 tablespoons fresh dill, chopped
- 1 clove garlic, minced
- Salt and black pepper, to taste

Instructions:

Preheat the oven to 375°F (190°C) and place salmon filets on a baking sheet. Drizzle olive oil over the salmon, sprinkle minced garlic evenly, and place lemon slices on top. Season with salt and black pepper. Bake for 15-20 minutes until the fish flakes easily. For the Lemon-Dill Sauce, whisk together Greek yogurt, lemon juice, chopped dill, minced garlic, salt, and black pepper. Serve the Baked Salmon with the Lemon-Dill Sauce drizzled over the top and garnish with fresh dill sprigs for added flavor. Enjoy this tender and healthy main course.

2. Grilled Shrimp and Avocado Salad

Ingredients:

For the Grilled Shrimp:

- 1 pound large shrimp, peeled and deveined
- 2 tablespoons olive oil
- 2 cloves garlic, minced
- 1 teaspoon paprika
- 1/2 teaspoon cayenne pepper
- Salt and black pepper, to taste
- Lemon wedges for serving

For the Salad:

- 4 cups mixed salad greens (e.g., lettuce, arugula, spinach)
- 2 ripe avocados, peeled, pitted, and sliced
- 1 cup cherry tomatoes, halved
- 1/2 red onion, thinly sliced
- 1/4 cup fresh cilantro or parsley, chopped

For the Lemon Vinaigrette:

- 1/4 cup extra-virgin olive oil
- 2 tablespoons fresh lemon juice
- 1 teaspoon Dijon mustard
- 1 clove garlic, minced
- Salt and black pepper, to taste

Instructions:

This recipe involves marinating grilled shrimp in olive oil, garlic, paprika, cayenne pepper, salt, and black pepper. After allowing the shrimp to sit for 15 minutes, grill them on skewers for 2-3 minutes per side until they turn pink and slightly charred. Remove the grilled shrimp and serve with lemon wedges. For the salad, combine mixed salad greens with sliced avocados, cherry tomatoes, thinly sliced red onion, and chopped cilantro or parsley. For the Lemon Vinaigrette, whisk together extra-virgin olive oil, fresh lemon juice, Dijon mustard, minced garlic, salt, and black pepper. Drizzle the vinaigrette over the salad and place the grilled shrimp on top. Serve the Grilled Shrimp and Avocado Salad as a refreshing main course, drizzling extra dressing over the shrimp and garnishing with fresh herbs.

3. Pan-Seared Tilapia with Mango Salsa

Ingredients:

For the Pan-Seared Tilapia:

- 4 tilapia filets
- 2 tablespoons olive oil
- 1 teaspoon paprika
- 1 teaspoon garlic powder
- Salt and black pepper, to taste
- Fresh lime wedges for serving

For the Mango Salsa:

- 2 ripe mangoes, peeled, pitted, and diced
- 1/2 red onion, finely chopped
- 1 red bell pepper, diced
- 1 jalapeño, seeded and finely chopped
- 1/4 cup fresh cilantro, chopped
- Juice of 1 lime
- Salt and black pepper, to taste

Instructions:

To prepare pan-seared tilapia, mix paprika, black pepper, salt, and garlic powder in a bowl. Coat each filet with the spice mixture and cook in olive oil for 3-4 minutes on each side until opaque. Squeeze fresh lime juice over the filets before serving. For the mango salsa, combine diced mangoes, jalapeño, cilantro, red onion, and red bell pepper. Add lime juice and adjust seasoning as needed. Present the pan-seared tilapia individually or on a tray, then top each filet with mango salsa. Garnish with more cilantro and serve with lime wedges. This quick and satisfying dinner is rich, vibrant, and light, making it a great choice for any meal.

4. Teriyaki Glazed Mahi-Mahi

Ingredients:

For the Teriyaki Glaze:

- 1/2 cup soy sauce
- 1/4 cup mirin (sweet rice wine)
- 2 tablespoons honey
- 1 tablespoon rice vinegar
- 1 teaspoon sesame oil
- 2 cloves garlic, minced
- 1 teaspoon fresh ginger, grated
- 1 tablespoon cornstarch (optional, for thickening)

For the Mahi-Mahi:

- 4 mahi-mahi filets
- Salt and black pepper, to taste
- 2 tablespoons vegetable oil
- Sesame seeds and chopped green onions for garnish (optional)

Instructions:

To make the Teriyaki Glaze, combine soy sauce, mirin, honey, rice vinegar, sesame oil, minced garlic, and grated ginger in a small saucepan. Simmer over medium heat, stirring occasionally to thicken the glaze. For a thicker glaze, mix cornstarch with water and stir into the teriyaki sauce. Set aside.

For the Mahi-Mahi, dry the filets and season them with salt and black pepper. Heat vegetable oil in a large skillet and sear the filets for 3-4 minutes per side until they develop a golden-brown crust and are cooked through. Pour the teriyaki glaze over the fish and allow it to cook for an additional 1-2 minutes.

Serve the Teriyaki Glazed Mahi on a serving platter, garnish with sesame seeds and chopped green onions, and serve over steamed rice or with side dishes. Enjoy this flavorful seafood dish.

5. Lemon Butter Cod with Asparagus

Ingredients:

For the Lemon Butter Cod:

- 4 cod filets
- Salt and black pepper, to taste
- 2 tablespoons olive oil
- 4 tablespoons unsalted butter
- 3 cloves garlic, minced
- Zest of 1 lemon
- Juice of 1 lemon
- 1 tablespoon fresh parsley, chopped

For the Asparagus:

- 1 bunch asparagus, ends trimmed
- 1 tablespoon olive oil
- Salt and black pepper, to taste
- Lemon wedges for serving

Instructions:

Preheat your oven to 375°F (190°C) and season cod filets with salt and black pepper. Heat olive oil in an oven-safe skillet and sear the cod for 2-3 minutes per side until they develop a golden-brown crust. Bake for an additional 8-10 minutes until cooked through and flakes easily. In the same skillet, add unsalted butter, minced garlic, lemon zest, lemon juice, and chopped parsley. Cook for 1-2 minutes to meld flavors and melt butter.

While the cod is baking, toss trimmed asparagus in olive oil, salt, and black pepper. Roast the asparagus for 10-12 minutes until tender but crisp. Serve the Lemon Butter Cod over roasted asparagus, spoon the lemon butter sauce over the cod filets, garnish with parsley, and serve with lemon wedges on the side. Enjoy this light and flavorful meal.

6. Tuna Nicoise Salad

Ingredients:

For the Salad:

- 2 cups baby potatoes, halved
- 4 large eggs
- 8 oz green beans, trimmed
- 2 cups cherry tomatoes, halved
- 1/2 red onion, thinly sliced
- 1/2 cup Niçoise olives
- 4 cups mixed salad greens
- 2 cans (5 oz each) tuna, drained

For the Vinaigrette:

- 1/4 cup red wine vinegar
- 1/2 cup extra-virgin olive oil
- 1 teaspoon Dijon mustard
- 1 clove garlic, minced
- Salt and black pepper, to taste

Instructions:

This recipe involves cooking baby potatoes in salted water until tender, then preparing eggs in a pot of boiling salted water. Blanch green beans in the same pot for 3-4 minutes until crisp-tender. Arrange the salad on a platter, top with cherry tomatoes, red onion, baby potatoes, hard-boiled eggs, green beans, Niçoise olives, and canned tuna. For the vinaigrette, whisk together red wine vinegar, extra-virgin olive oil, Dijon mustard, minced garlic, salt, and black pepper. Drizzle the vinaigrette over the salad just before serving, or serve additional on the side. Gently toss the salad, ensuring it's well-coated with the vinaigrette, and serve immediately for a refreshing and satisfying meal.

7. Poached Halibut with Garlic and Herb Butter

Ingredients:

For the Poached Halibut:

- 4 halibut filets
- Salt and black pepper, to taste
- 2 tablespoons olive oil
- 1 cup dry white wine
- 1 lemon, sliced
- 4 sprigs fresh thyme

For the Garlic and Herb Butter:

- 1/2 cup unsalted butter, softened
- 3 cloves garlic, minced
- 2 tablespoons fresh parsley, chopped
- 1 tablespoon fresh chives, chopped
- Salt and black pepper, to taste

Instructions:

To make poached halibut, season the filets with salt and black pepper, heat olive oil in a pan, and sear until golden-brown. Add lemon slices, white wine, and fresh thyme sprigs. Simmer for 8-10 minutes until the fish is opaque and flakes easily. Cover and pouch. In a separate bowl, mix melted unsalted butter, minced garlic, parsley, chives, salt, and black pepper. Place the poached filets on serving dishes, drizzle with the herb and garlic butter, and add more herbs as a garnish. Serve immediately for a refined seafood meal. This elegant and delectable dish is sure to impress.

CHAPTER 4: SATISFYING SIDES AND SNACKS

A. Guilt-free Snacking

1. Blueberry and Almond Yogurt Parfait

Ingredients:

- Greek yogurt
- Fresh blueberries
- Sliced almonds
- Honey

Instructions:

This recipe involves layering Greek yogurt, fresh blueberries, sliced almonds, honey, and almonds in a glass or dish. The yogurt is then topped with almonds for sweetness. The mixture is then topped with honey and almond sprinkles. The yogurt and almond parfait is a healthy and visually appealing breakfast or snack, made with creamy yogurt, crunchy almonds, sweet blueberries, and honey. The process is repeated until the parfait is full.

2. Avocado and Tomato Salsa with Whole Grain Crackers

Ingredients:

- Ripe avocados, diced
- Cherry tomatoes, diced
- Red onion, finely chopped
- Fresh cilantro, chopped
- Lime juice
- Salt and black pepper, to taste
- Whole grain crackers

Instructions:

This recipe involves combining diced avocados, cherry tomatoes, red onion, and fresh cilantro in a bowl. Lime juice is added for a zesty flavor, and salt and black pepper are added for taste. The mixture is gently tossed to ensure even distribution. The salsa is then served with whole grain crackers for a satisfying snack. The creamy avocado, juicy tomatoes, and refreshing cilantro make for a delightful and nutritious treat.

3. Cucumber and Hummus Bites

Ingredients:

- English cucumbers, sliced into rounds
- Hummus
- Cherry tomatoes, halved
- Fresh dill, for garnish (optional)

Instructions:

Cut English cucumbers into rounds for a sturdy bite. Top each cucumber slice with a dollop of hummus, halved cherry tomato, and a fresh dill garnish. Transfer the bites to a plate for presentation. Serve as a healthy starter or snack, enjoying the sharpness of the cucumber, creaminess of the hummus, and the flavor explosion of the cherry tomatoes. Enjoy every mouthful.

4. Quinoa and Berry Protein Balls

Ingredients:

- Cooked quinoa, cooled
- Mixed berries (blueberries, raspberries)
- Almond butter
- Chia seeds
- Honey

Instructions:

This recipe involves combining cooked quinoa with mixed berries, almond butter, chia seeds, honey, and chia seeds in a bowl. The mixture is then mixed thoroughly, rolled into bite-sized balls, and placed on a tray or plate. The balls are then refrigerated for at least 30 minutes to firm up. These protein-packed and flavorful balls can be served as a nutritious snack or energy boost, and the combination of quinoa, berries, and almond butter is a tasty and wholesome treat.

5. Spinach and Artichoke Stuffed Mushrooms

Ingredients:

- Large mushrooms, cleaned and stems removed
- Fresh spinach, chopped
- Artichoke hearts, chopped
- Feta cheese, crumbled
- Garlic, minced

Instructions:

Preheat the oven to 375°F (190°C). Mix spinach, artichoke hearts, feta cheese, and garlic in a bowl. Clean and remove mushrooms. Stuff each mushroom cap with the spinach and artichoke mixture, pressing gently. Place on a baking sheet and bake for 15-20 minutes until tender and golden. Cool slightly before serving. Garnish with more feta and parsley. Serve as a nutritious appetizer or side dish, enjoying the rich combination of spinach, artichoke, and feta.

6. *Turmeric and Ginger Roasted Chickpeas*

Ingredients:

- Canned chickpeas, drained and rinsed
- Olive oil
- Ground turmeric
- Ground ginger
- Smoked paprika
- Salt

Instructions:

Preheat the oven to 400°F (200°C). Rinse and drain canned chickpeas, then coat them with olive oil. Sprinkle ground turmeric, ginger, smoked paprika, and salt over the chickpeas, adjusting the amounts to your taste. Toss the chickpeas again to ensure they are evenly coated. Spread the seasoned chickpeas on a baking sheet and roast in the oven for 25-30 minutes, shaking the pan halfway. Once golden and crispy, remove from the oven and let them cool slightly. Serve the Turmeric and Ginger Roasted Chickpeas as a crunchy, flavorful snack.

B. Healthy Dips and Spreads

1. Roasted Red Pepper Hummus

Ingredients:

- 1 can (15 oz) chickpeas, drained and rinsed
- 1/2 cup roasted red peppers, drained
- 1/4 cup tahini
- 2 cloves garlic, minced
- 2 tablespoons olive oil
- 1 tablespoon lemon juice
- 1/2 teaspoon ground cumin
- Salt and black pepper, to taste

Instructions:

This recipe involves blending chickpeas, tahini, garlic, roasted red peppers, olive oil, lemon juice, ground cumin, salt, and black pepper in a food processor. It's then pureed until smooth, adding water as needed. The spices are adjusted as needed. The hummus is then spooned onto a serving dish, drizzled with olive oil, and topped with fresh parsley or paprika. It pairs well with crackers, vegetable sticks, or pita bread. This homemade hummus is a delicious and nutritious dip.

2. Greek Yogurt Tzatziki

Ingredients:

- 1 cup Greek yogurt
- 1 cucumber, finely grated and drained
- 2 cloves garlic, minced
- 1 tablespoon fresh dill, chopped
- 1 tablespoon extra-virgin olive oil
- 1 teaspoon lemon juice
- Salt and black pepper, to taste

Instructions:

This recipe involves combining Greek yogurt, cucumber, garlic, dill, extra-virgin olive oil, and lemon juice in a bowl. Season with salt and black pepper, then taste and adjust the flavors. Refrigerate for at least 30 minutes to allow flavors to meld. Before serving, stir the mixture and drizzle with olive oil. This Greek Yogurt Tzatziki can be served as a dip with pita bread, vegetable sticks, or as a condiment for grilled meats. Enjoy the cool and tangy flavor of this homemade dish.

3. Avocado and Edamame Spread

Ingredients:

- 1 ripe avocado
- 1 cup edamame, cooked and shelled
- 1 clove garlic, minced
- 2 tablespoons fresh cilantro, chopped
- 1 tablespoon lime juice
- Salt and black pepper, to taste

Instructions:

This recipe involves blending cooked edamame, fresh cilantro, lime juice, minced garlic, and ripe avocado in a food processor until a creamy, smooth consistency is achieved. Adjust seasoning with salt and black pepper, then pulse to mix in spices. Adjust consistency by adding water or olive oil if needed. Spoon the spread onto a serving dish and garnish with cilantro or lime zest for freshness.

Serve as a dip for veggie sticks, toast, or whole grain crackers, or enjoy as a nutritious snack or appetizer.

4. Spinach and Kale Pesto

Ingredients:

- 2 cups fresh spinach leaves
- 1 cup fresh kale leaves, stems removed
- 1/2 cup walnuts or pine nuts, toasted
- 1/2 cup grated Parmesan cheese
- 2 cloves garlic, peeled
- 1/2 cup extra-virgin olive oil
- Juice of 1 lemon
- Salt and black pepper, to taste

Instructions:

This recipe involves blending spinach, kale, toasted nuts, grated Parmesan cheese, and peeled garlic in a food processor. The ingredients are then pulsed until finely chopped. The pesto is then added to the mixture, and the lemon juice is added. The pesto is then tasted and seasoned with salt and black pepper. If the pesto is too thick, more olive oil can be added. The pesto is then transferred to a jar or bowl for serving. Optional toppings include extra Parmesan cheese or fresh basil. This nutrient-rich pesto can be served over pasta, spread on sandwiches, or as a dip for vegetable crudites.

5. Sun-Dried Tomato and Basil Tapenade

Ingredients:

- 1 cup sun-dried tomatoes (dry-packed), rehydrated and drained
- 1/2 cup fresh basil leaves
- 1/4 cup black olives, pitted
- 2 cloves garlic, minced
- 1/4 cup extra-virgin olive oil
- 1 tablespoon balsamic vinegar
- Salt and black pepper, to taste

Instructions:

This recipe involves blending rehydrated sun-dried tomatoes, basil leaves, pitted black olives, and minced garlic in a food processor. The ingredients are then pulsed until a coarse paste is formed. The extra-virgin olive oil is gradually added, and the balsamic vinegar is added. The tapenade is then tasted and seasoned with salt and black pepper. If too thick, more olive oil is added. The tapenade is then transferred to a serving bowl and garnished with fresh basil leaves or olive oil. It can be served with crusty bread, crackers, or as a condiment for grilled vegetables or meats.

6. *Walnut and Roasted Garlic White Bean Dip*

Ingredients:

- 1 can (15 oz) white beans, drained and rinsed
- 1/2 cup walnuts, toasted
- 1 head of garlic, roasted
- 2 tablespoons lemon juice
- 1/4 cup extra-virgin olive oil
- Salt and black pepper, to taste
- Fresh parsley, chopped (for garnish)

Instructions:

Preheat the oven to 400°F (200°C). Roast garlic cloves in the oven for 30-40 minutes until soft and golden. In a food processor, combine white beans, toasted walnuts, roasted garlic cloves, and lemon juice. Pulse until coarsely chopped. Slowly drizzle extra-virgin olive oil into the mixture until it reaches a smooth consistency. Season with salt and black pepper to taste. If too thick, add more olive oil. Transfer the dip to a serving bowl and garnish with fresh parsley for color. Serve this flavorful and nutty dip with pita bread, vegetable sticks, or as a spread for sandwiches. Enjoy the rich and creamy goodness of this Walnut and Roasted Garlic White Bean Dip as a healthy snack.

C. Wholesome Side Dishes

1. *Quinoa and Vegetable Pilaf*

Ingredients:

- 1 cup quinoa, rinsed
- 2 cups vegetable broth
- 1 tablespoon olive oil
- 1 onion, finely chopped
- 2 carrots, diced
- 1 zucchini, diced
- 1 red bell pepper, diced
- 2 cloves garlic, minced
- 1 teaspoon ground cumin
- 1 teaspoon ground coriander
- Salt and black pepper, to taste
- Fresh parsley, chopped (for garnish)

Instructions:

This recipe involves preparing a Quinoa and Vegetable Pilaf. Rinse the quinoa in cold water and cook it in vegetable broth for 15-20 minutes until tender. Heat olive oil in a large pan over medium heat and add onion slices. Sauté red bell pepper, carrots, and zucchini in a skillet until crisp-tender. Add ground coriander, cumin, and garlic and fry for another minute. Once done, add the quinoa and sautéed veggies to the pan and fluff it with a fork. Season with salt and black pepper to taste and adjust seasonings as needed. Sprinkle freshly chopped parsley on top of the pilaf. Serve this dish as a light main course or side dish, enjoying the nutrient-rich blend of colorful veggies and quinoa.

2. Roasted Brussels Sprouts with Balsamic Glaze

Ingredients:

- 1 pound Brussels sprouts, trimmed and halved
- 2 tablespoons olive oil
- Salt and black pepper, to taste
- 2 tablespoons balsamic glaze (store-bought or homemade)

Instructions:

Preheat the oven to 400°F or 200°C. Coat Brussels sprouts in olive oil, salt, and black pepper. Arrange them on a baking sheet and roast for 20-25 minutes until crispy and golden brown. Remove from the oven and serve on a platter. Drizzle balsamic glaze over the sprouts while they're still warm. Add more salt and pepper to taste. Serve as a side dish with the roasted Brussels sprouts, enjoying the caramelized sweetness of the glaze. Enjoy the delicious and nourishing combination of flavors and textures.

3. *Cauliflower Mash with Garlic and Herbs*

Ingredients:

- 1 large head cauliflower, cut into florets
- 2 cloves garlic, minced
- 2 tablespoons olive oil
- 1/4 cup fresh parsley, chopped
- Salt and black pepper, to taste
- 1/4 cup grated Parmesan cheese (optional)

Instructions:

To make a cauliflower mash, steam or boil cauliflower florets until tender. In a large bowl, combine steamed cauliflower, minced garlic, olive oil, and fresh parsley. Blend the ingredients until smooth and creamy, or mash with a potato masher for a chunkier texture. Season with salt and black pepper, and add grated Parmesan cheese for richness. Transfer the mashed cauliflower to a serving bowl and garnish with parsley. This cauliflower mash is a low-carb alternative to traditional mashed potatoes and is a delicious and nutritious side dish.

4. Lemon Herb Couscous Salad

Ingredients:

- 1 cup couscous
- 1 1/4 cups vegetable broth or water
- Zest and juice of 1 lemon
- 2 tablespoons extra-virgin olive oil
- 1/4 cup fresh parsley, chopped
- 1/4 cup fresh mint, chopped
- 1/4 cup feta cheese, crumbled
- Salt and black pepper, to taste

Instructions:

To make a Lemon Herb Couscous Salad, boil water or vegetable broth, add couscous, and wait five minutes. Separate the grains, then mix cooked couscous, extra-virgin olive oil, lemon zest, and juice in a bowl. Add mint and fresh parsley, and mix well. Gently mix in feta cheese crumbles. Season with black pepper and salt, and adjust seasonings as needed. Let the salad cool in the fridge for at least half an hour before serving. This light main meal or side dish can be enjoyed with its crisp, zesty aromas and fluffy texture.

5. Grilled Asparagus with Lemon Zest

Ingredients:

- 1 bunch fresh asparagus, trimmed
- 2 tablespoons olive oil
- Zest of 1 lemon
- Salt and black pepper, to taste
- Lemon wedges (for serving)

Instructions:

Preheat a grill or grill pan over medium-high heat. Toss trimmed asparagus with olive oil and arrange on the grill. Grill for 3-5 minutes, turning occasionally, until tender and with grill marks. Transfer to a serving platter. Sprinkle lemon zest over the asparagus while still warm. Season with salt and black pepper to taste. Serve with lemon wedges on the side. Enjoy the smoky grill flavor, fresh lemon zest, and crisp asparagus. This dish is a delightful and healthy side that complements various main courses.

6. Mango and Black Bean Salsa

Ingredients:

- 1 ripe mango, peeled, pitted, and diced
- 1 can (15 oz) black beans, drained and rinsed
- 1 red bell pepper, diced
- 1/2 red onion, finely chopped
- 1 jalapeño, seeds removed and finely chopped
- Juice of 2 limes
- 2 tablespoons fresh cilantro, chopped
- Salt and black pepper, to taste
- Tortilla chips (for serving)

Instructions:

This recipe involves combining diced mango, black beans, red bell pepper, red onion, and jalapeño in a large bowl. Lime juice is added to the mixture, along with fresh cilantro. Season with salt and black pepper, and gently mix. Allow the salsa to sit for a few minutes to meld flavors. Serve with tortilla chips for dipping. This vibrant salsa is perfect for snacking, topping grilled chicken or fish, or as a side dish for summer gatherings. Enjoy the sweet and savory combination of mango and black beans.

CHAPTER 5: DESSERTS FOR AGELESS BLISS

A. Indulgent Yet Healthy Desserts

1. Dark Chocolate Avocado Mousse

Ingredients:

- Ripe avocados
- Unsweetened cocoa powder
- Maple syrup or honey
- Vanilla extract
- Pinch of sea salt

Instructions:

Blend ripe avocados, unsweetened cocoa powder, maple syrup, honey, vanilla extract, and sea salt in a food processor. Chill the mousse in the refrigerator for at least an hour before serving. Garnish with berries or cocoa powder for an extra touch. Enjoy this guilt-free dessert with anti-aging benefits.

2. Berry Chia Seed Pudding

Ingredients:

- Chia seeds
- Almond milk
- Honey or agave syrup
- Mixed berries (strawberries, blueberries, raspberries)
- Unsweetened coconut flakes

Instructions:

Firstly,chia seeds, almond milk, and honey or agave syrup are combined in a dish. Refrigerate the mixture for at least 4 hours or overnight to absorb the liquid, creating a pudding-like consistency. Stir the mixture before serving to ensure uniform texture. Arrange mixed berries on top of the pudding, adding unsweetened coconut flakes for extra texture and sweetness. Sprinkle more honey or agave syrup for added sweetness. Serve the cooled Berry Chia Seed Pudding, a guilt-free, healthy dessert that combines the taste of mixed berries with the health benefits of chia seeds.

3. Greek Yogurt Parfait with Granola and Berries

Ingredients:

- Greek yogurt
- Granola (choose a low-sugar option)
- Mixed berries (strawberries, blueberries, raspberries)
- Honey

Instructions:

In a glass or dish, arrange the Greek yogurt, granola, mixed berries, honey, and berries in layers according to this recipe. Evenly distribute the yogurt, then top with the granola, mixed berries, and honey. After that, sprinkle the berries on top of the yogurt and drizzle with honey for sweetness. Up to the top, the layers are repeated, then berries are placed on top. Honey is an optional addition for sweetness. The parfait, which combines the smoothness of Greek yogurt, the crunch of granola, and the sweetness of fresh berries, is served immediately. This is a nutritious diet choice that fights aging.

4. Baked Apples with Cinnamon and Walnuts

Ingredients:

- Apples (choose a sweet variety like Honeycrisp or Fuji)
- Coconut oil (or melted butter)
- Ground cinnamon
- Chopped walnuts
- Honey

Instructions:

To make a delicious apple dessert, preheat the oven to 375°F or 190°C. Wash and core the apples, leaving the bottoms whole. In a small bowl, combine ground cinnamon and melted coconut oil. Transfer the cores to a baking tray and apply the cinnamon-scented oil mixture. Blend chopped walnuts and honey in another bowl. Stuff the honeyed walnut mixture into each cored apple. Bake for 20-25 minutes until soft but not mushy. Allow the apples to cool before serving. Sprinkle more honey over the cooked apples before serving. Serve warm with walnuts and cinnamon for a cozy dessert that enhances the natural sweetness of apples and amplifies their flavor.

5. Coconut and Mango Chia Seed Popsicles

Ingredients:

- Chia seeds
- Coconut milk
- Ripe mango, pureed
- Honey or agave syrup

Instructions:

To make Chia Seed Popsicles, blend coconut milk and chia seeds in a dish. Refrigerate the mixture for several hours or overnight to absorb the coconut milk. Layer pureed ripe mango with the chia pudding mixture in popsicle molds, placing a popsicle stick inside each mold. Freeze the popsicles for at least 4-6 hours, then remove them from the molds. Pour honey or agave syrup over the frozen popsicles before serving. Enjoy the richness of chia seeds, the sweetness of ripe mango, and the creaminess of coconut in this tropical treat, a tasty and nutritious way to cool down while indulging in dessert.

B. Fruit-Forward Sweet Treats

1. Tropical Fruit Salad with Mint Infusion

Ingredients:

- Pineapple, diced
- Mango, diced
- Kiwi, sliced
- Strawberries, sliced
- Fresh mint leaves, finely chopped
- Lime juice
- Honey or agave syrup (optional)

Instructions:

In a large bowl, combine diced mango, pineapple, strawberries, and kiwi. Drizzle lime juice and mint leaves over the tropical fruits, then mix thoroughly. Add honey or agave syrup for sweetness. Refrigerate for at least half an hour to allow flavors to mingle. Gently mix the fruit salad before serving. This colorful and refreshing fruit salad is perfect for a hot day snack or dessert. It combines the tropical richness of mango and pineapple with the zesty lime and the cool touch of mint, making it an ideal choice for a refreshing and colorful meal.

2. Honey-Lime Grilled Pineapple

Ingredients:

- Fresh pineapple, peeled, cored, and cut into spears or rings
- Honey
- Lime juice
- Fresh mint leaves, chopped (optional)
- Vanilla ice cream or Greek yogurt (optional, for serving)

Instructions:

To prepare a delicious grilled pineapple, heat the grill to medium-high and prepare a marinade by mixing lime juice and honey. Brush the pineapple rings or spears with the honey-lime marinade, then cook for two to three minutes on each side until caramelized and grill marks appear. For extra flavor, baste the pineapple with extra marinade. Transfer the grilled pineapple to a plate and serve with chopped fresh mint for a fresh touch. Serve it alone or with Greek yogurt or vanilla ice cream for an added treat. Enjoy the acidic and sweet flavors of the pineapple, a sweet delicacy that embodies summertime simplicity and joy.

3. Mixed Berry Frozen Yogurt Bark

Ingredients:

- Greek yogurt

- Mixed berries (strawberries, blueberries, raspberries)
- Honey or maple syrup
- Granola (optional)

Instructions:

Create a Mixed Berry Frozen Yogurt Bark by combining Greek yogurt, honey or maple syrup, and mixed berries. Line a baking sheet with parchment paper and create a thin layer of yogurt. Gently press mixed berries into the yogurt layer. Optionally, top with granola for crunch. Freeze the yogurt bark for three to four hours until it solidifies. Once frozen, split it into manageable pieces and serve as a cool and healthy frozen treat. Enjoy the crunch of granola, sweet mixed berries, and creamy Greek yogurt in this tasty and healthy frozen snack.

4. Citrus Mint Sorbet Cups

Ingredients:

- Orange juice
- Lemon juice
- Lime juice
- Fresh mint leaves, chopped
- Agave syrup or honey
- Fresh citrus slices (for garnish)

Instructions:

In a bowl, mix lime, lemon, and orange juices with chopped mint leaves. Add honey or agave syrup to taste. Transfer the mixture to serving mugs or molds and freeze until solidified. Top each cup with fresh citrus segments for a pop of color. Serve as a refreshing dessert or a refreshing refreshing drink to round off a dinner. Enjoy the spicy and minty citrus sorbet, perfect for a refreshing and revitalizing finish to a cool dinner.

5. Roasted Peach with Balsamic Glaze

Ingredients:

- Ripe peaches, halved and pitted
- Olive oil
- Balsamic glaze
- Honey
- Fresh thyme leaves (optional)

Instructions:

Place the pitted and halved peaches on a baking sheet and preheat the oven to 375°F (190°C). Drizzle the peaches with olive oil, then roast them for 15 to 20 minutes, or until they are soft and caramelized. While roasting, reheat a balsamic glaze in a small pot over low heat. After transferring the peaches to a serving tray, pour the honey and glaze over them. For a fragrant touch, feel free to add some fresh thyme leaves on top. Enjoy the roasted peaches' sweet and tart tastes while serving warm. This is a classy but elegant dessert that perfectly embodies summer.

C. Decadent Chocolate Creations

1. Dark Chocolate Raspberry Avocado Truffles

Ingredients:

- Ripe avocados
- Dark chocolate, melted
- Fresh raspberries
- Cocoa powder (for rolling)
- Honey or maple syrup (optional, for extra sweetness)
- Chopped nuts or shredded coconut (optional, for coating)

Instructions:

To make Dark Chocolate Raspberry Avocado Truffles, mash ripe avocados until smooth. Melt dark chocolate in a double boiler or microwave, then fold in the avocado mixture. Add honey or maple syrup for sweetness. Place a fresh raspberry in the center of your palm and form a truffle shape. Roll each truffle in cocoa powder or shredded coconut or chopped almonds for a textural boost. Chill the truffles for one to two hours or until they solidify. Enjoy these decadent and healthy truffles, which combine the creamy texture of avocado, the richness of dark chocolate, and the crispness of raspberries. Enjoy these decadent and healthy truffles when they're cold.

2. Chocolate Avocado Mousse with Sea Salt

Ingredients:

- Ripe avocados
- Dark chocolate, melted
- Cocoa powder
- Maple syrup or honey
- Vanilla extract
- Pinch of sea salt
- Fresh berries (for garnish, optional)

Instructions:

This recipe involves blending ripe avocados, dark chocolate, cocoa powder, honey or maple syrup, and vanilla extract in a food processor or blender until creamy and smooth. Adjust sweetness with additional honey or maple syrup. Add a pinch of sea salt and blend again. Pour the chocolate and avocado mousse into bowls or serving glasses, optionally adding toppings or fresh berries. Chill in the fridge for at least two hours to solidify. Present the cooled chocolate avocado mousse topped with sea salt, enjoying the luscious, creamy chocolate mousse made possible by avocados and the sweet and salty taste of sea salt.

3. Double Chocolate Banana Bread

Ingredients:

- Ripe bananas, mashed
- All-purpose flour
- Cocoa powder
- Baking soda
- Salt
- Unsalted butter, melted
- Brown sugar
- Eggs
- Vanilla extract
- Greek yogurt

- Dark chocolate chips or chunks

Instructions:

To make a delicious Double Chocolate Banana Bread, set the oven to 175°C/350°F and oil and dust a loaf pan. In a mixing bowl, blend mashed ripe bananas, brown sugar, eggs, melted butter, and vanilla essence. In another bowl, combine flour, baking soda, cocoa powder, and salt. Stir the dry ingredients into the banana mixture until smooth, then gradually add Greek yogurt. Gently fold in dark chocolate chips, saving some for the topping. Transfer the mixture to the loaf pan and level the top. Top with the reserved dark chocolate chips. Bake for 55-65 minutes or until a toothpick inserted in the middle comes out clean. After cooling, slice and enjoy the rich and moist banana bread with two servings of chocolate delight.

4. Chocolate-Covered Strawberries with Almond Butter Drizzle

Ingredients:

- Fresh strawberries, washed and dried
- Dark chocolate, melted
- Almond butter
- Chopped almonds (optional, for garnish)

Instructions:

To make a chocolate-covered strawberry dessert, line a tray or dish with parchment paper. Melt dark chocolate in a double boiler or microwave until smooth. Dip each strawberry into the melted chocolate, then transfer them to the prepared dish. Heat almond butter in a microwave-safe bowl until slightly runny, then pour it on top of the chocolate-coated strawberries. Optionally, top with chopped almonds for extra crunch. Refrigerate the tray for 15-20 minutes to set the chocolate coating. Once hardened, transfer the chocolate-covered strawberries to a dish for presentation. Enjoy these decadent confections, blending dark chocolate, almond butter, and strawberry sweetness.

5. Mint Chocolate Chip Chia Seed Pudding

Ingredients:

- Chia seeds
- Almond milk (or any milk of choice)
- Peppermint extract
- Maple syrup or agave syrup
- Dark chocolate chips
- Fresh mint leaves (for garnish, optional)

Instructions:

Chia seeds, almond milk, peppermint essence, and maple syrup are combined to make a tasty and nutritious treat known as chia seed pudding. To allow the liquid to soak, place it in the refrigerator for at least four hours or overnight. Stir the pudding and spread the dark chocolate chunks equally after serving. Add some mint leaves as a garnish for a refreshing pop. Enjoy the cool blend of mint, dark chocolate chips, and almond milk as you serve the pudding in separate cups or bowls.

D. Dairy-Free Delights

1. Coconut Mango Nice Cream

Ingredients:

- Ripe mangoes, peeled, pitted, and chopped
- Coconut cream or full-fat coconut milk
- Unsweetened shredded coconut
- Maple syrup or agave syrup (optional, for added sweetness)
- Toasted coconut flakes (for garnish, optional)

Instructions:

Chop mangoes and freeze them for 2-3 hours. In a blender, blend frozen mango chunks, coconut cream, and unsweetened shredded coconut until smooth and creamy. Add maple syrup or agave syrup if desired. Transfer the mixture to a bowl and optionally fold in additional shredded coconut for texture. If a firmer texture is desired, freeze for an additional 1-2 hours. Serve the Coconut Mango Nice Cream in bowls or cones and garnish with toasted coconut flakes for added flavor. This tropical and dairy-free dessert combines mango's lusciousness with coconut's creamy richness, making it a refreshing and guilt-free dessert option.

2. Almond Milk Chocolate Pudding

Ingredients:

- 2 cups almond milk
- 1/2 cup granulated sugar
- 1/4 cup unsweetened cocoa powder
- 1/4 cup cornstarch
- 1/4 teaspoon salt
- 1 teaspoon vanilla extract
- Dark chocolate chips (optional, for garnish)
- Sliced almonds (optional, for garnish)

Instructions:

In a medium-sized pot, combine sugar, cornstarch, cocoa powder, and salt. Gradually add almond milk to the dry ingredients, stirring to prevent lumps. Bring the mixture to a moderate boil, then reduce heat to a simmer and whisk for two to three minutes. Turn off heat and mix in vanilla extract. Transfer the chocolate pudding to separate dishes or serving cups, let it cool, cover, and refrigerate for at least two hours. If desired, top with sliced almonds and dark chocolate chips before serving. This decadent, dairy-free chocolate pudding is perfect for chocolate lovers.

3. Vegan Chocolate Chip Cookies

Ingredients:

- 1 cup all-purpose flour
- 1/2 teaspoon baking soda
- 1/4 teaspoon salt
- 1/4 cup coconut oil, melted
- 1/2 cup brown sugar, packed
- 1/4 cup granulated sugar
- 1 teaspoon vanilla extract
- 3 tablespoons unsweetened applesauce
- 1 cup vegan chocolate chips

Instructions:

Preheat the oven to 350°F (175°C) and line a baking sheet with parchment paper. In a bowl, whisk together flour, baking soda, and salt. In a separate bowl, mix melted coconut oil, brown sugar, granulated sugar, and vanilla extract. Add applesauce to the wet ingredients and mix until smooth. Gradually add dry ingredients to the wet ingredients, stir until it is well combined and fold in vegan chocolate chips. Drop rounded tablespoons of cookie dough onto the baking sheet, leaving space between each cookie. Bake in the oven for 10-12 minutes or until golden brown. Allow cookies to cool on the baking sheet before transferring them to a wire rack to cool completely. Store the cookies in an airtight container. Enjoy these delicious vegan chocolate chip cookies, satisfying your sweet tooth in a plant-based way.

4. Cashew Vanilla Bean Ice Cream

Ingredients:

- 2 cups raw cashews, soaked overnight and drained
- 1 can (14 ounces) full-fat coconut milk
- 1/2 cup maple syrup or agave syrup

- 1 vanilla bean, scraped (or 2 teaspoons vanilla extract)
- Pinch of salt

Instructions:

To make a dairy-free Cashew Vanilla Bean Ice Cream, blend soaked cashews, coconut milk, maple syrup, vanilla bean, and salt. Blend until smooth and creamy and adjust sweetness by adding more maple or agave syrup as needed. Fill an ice cream machine with the cashew mixture and churn it to a soft-serve consistency. Freeze the partially churned ice cream for at least 4 hours until solidified. Allow it to soften slightly at room temperature before serving. Enjoy the nutty and velvety vegan ice cream, which can be garnished with fresh fruit, chopped nuts, or a drizzle of maple syrup. Enjoy the smooth and creamy texture of this delicious dairy-free treat.

5. Chia Seed Coconut Milk Rice Pudding

Ingredients:

- 1 cup Arborio rice
- 2 cans (27 ounces) coconut milk
- 1/2 cup sugar
- 1 teaspoon vanilla extract

- 1/2 cup chia seeds
- Fresh berries or tropical fruit (for topping, optional)
- Shredded coconut (for garnish, optional)

Instructions:

Rinse Arborio rice and combine it with coconut milk, sugar, and vanilla extract in a medium-sized saucepan. Simmer gently for 25-30 minutes until the rice is cooked and the mixture thickens. Remove from heat and stir in chia seeds. Cool for a few minutes. Transfer the pudding to serving bowls or glasses and refrigerate for at least 2 hours. Gently stir the pudding before serving. Optionally, top with fresh berries or tropical fruit and garnish with shredded coconut for texture. Enjoy this creamy, coconut-infused rice pudding with a tropical twist, making it a delightful and satisfying dessert.

CHAPTER 6: BEVERAGES FOR ETERNAL YOUTH

A. Hydration and Anti-Aging Elixirs

1. Radiant Berry Infusion Elixir

Ingredients:

- Mixed berries (such as blueberries, raspberries, strawberries)
- Fresh mint leaves
- Water
- Optional: Honey or agave syrup for sweetness

Instructions:

To create a radiant berry infusion elixir, wash mixed berries and chop larger fruits like strawberries into smaller pieces. In a pitcher or container, add mixed berries and mint leaves, fill with water, and add honey or agave syrup for sweetness. Stir gently and refrigerate for 2-4 hours or overnight to let flavors infuse. Strain the mixture to remove berries and mint leaves, and serve over ice for a refreshing, antioxidant-rich drink. This elixir promotes radiant skin and overall well-being, and adjusts sweetness to your preference.

2. Tropical Citrus Hydrator Elixir

Ingredients:

- 1 orange, sliced
- 1 lime, sliced
- 1 lemon, sliced
- 2-3 slices of fresh pineapple
- Fresh mint leaves
- Coconut water or regular water
- Ice cubes

Instructions:

This recipe involves preparing citrus fruits, pineapple slices, and mint leaves. In a container, combine the fruits, pineapple, and mint leaves. Fill the container with coconut water or regular water, add ice cubes, stir gently, and let it sit in the refrigerator for 1-2 hours. When ready to serve, pour the tropical citrus hydrator elixir into glasses over ice. Garnish each glass with a slice of citrus fruit or mint for visual appeal. This refreshing beverage is perfect for staying hydrated while enjoying a burst of tropical goodness. Adjust the sweetness and intensity by varying the fruit slices for a tropical treat.

3. Blueberry Lavender Vitality Elixir

Ingredients:

- 1 cup fresh or frozen blueberries
- 2-3 sprigs of fresh lavender (or 1-2 teaspoons of dried culinary lavender)
- Honey or agave syrup (optional)
- Water
- Ice cubes

Instructions:

This recipe involves rinsing fresh blueberries and combining them with lavender sprigs in a saucepan. The mixture is then simmered until the blueberries burst and release their flavor and color. After cooling, strain the liquid through cheesecloth or a fine-mesh sieve to remove particles. Honey or agave syrup can be added to sweeten the elixir. The elixir should be left in the fridge for at least 60 minutes. Glasses with ice should be filed and served. For a visually appealing presentation, floating blueberries or a fresh lavender stem can be added. This refreshing beverage combines antioxidants from blueberries with the relaxing scent of lavender, offering a refreshing and calming beverage with potential health benefits. Adjust the sweetness to suit individual tastes.

4. Pomegranate Green Tea Reviver Elixir

Ingredients:

- 2 green tea bags
- 1 cup pomegranate juice (unsweetened)
- Fresh mint leaves
- Honey or agave syrup (optional)
- Water
- Ice cubes

Instructions:

To make a Pomegranate Green Tea Reviver Elixir, boil water, place tea bags in a heat proof container, steep for 3-5 minutes, and let cool. Add pomegranate juice, honey or agave syrup, and mint leaves for extra flavor. Refrigerate for 1-2 hours to blend flavors. Serve in glasses over ice and garnish with mint or pomegranate arils for a decorative touch. This elixir offers antioxidants from green tea and tangy sweetness from pomegranate juice, making it a revitalizing and refreshing drink. Adjust sweetness and mint intensity to your preference for a refreshing and hydrating drink.

5. *Peach Chamomile Glow Elixir*

Ingredients:

- 2-3 ripe peaches, sliced (or 1 cup of frozen peach slices)
- 2-3 chamomile tea bags
- Honey or agave syrup (optional)
- Water
- Ice cubes

Instructions:

To make a Peach Chamomile Glow Elixir, cut ripe peaches in half, remove the pits, and thaw them gently if frozen. Fill a pot with boiling water and transfer chamomile tea bags into a heat-resistant container. Infuse the chamomile flavor by pouring boiling water over the tea bags and allowing them to soak for five to seven minutes. After allowing the tea to cool, add the sliced peaches to the pitcher and gently mash them. If desired, add honey or agave syrup to sweeten the elixir. Refrigerate the elixir for at least an hour to allow flavors to combine. Pour the Peach Chamomile Glow Elixir into glasses with ice and add a peach slice or fresh chamomile rim for an eye-catching presentation. This delicious and soothing drink combines the natural sweetness of peaches with the calming aroma of chamomile.

B. Skin-Glowing Smoothie Bowls

1. Berry Burst Radiance Bowl

Ingredients:

- 1 cup mixed berries (strawberries, blueberries, raspberries)
- 1 ripe banana, sliced
- 1/2 cup Greek yogurt or dairy-free alternative
- 2 tablespoons honey or maple syrup (optional for added sweetness)
- 1/4 cup granola or nuts/seeds for crunch
- Fresh mint leaves for garnish (optional)

Instructions:

Wash berries and cut bananas to prepare a Berry Burst Radiance Bowl. Blend together granola, Greek yogurt, honey/maple syrup, banana slices, berries, and till smooth. Transfer into a bowl, add granola, almonds, or seeds for crunch, and add mint leaves for color. Savor it as a filling breakfast or snack, or add more richness by modifying it with nut butter, superfood toppings, or other fruits.

2. *Mango Turmeric Sunshine Bowl*

Ingredients:

- 1 ½ cups frozen mango chunks
- 1 ripe banana
- ½ tsp ground turmeric
- ½ cup Greek yogurt or coconut yogurt
- ½ cup orange juice (freshly squeezed or store-bought)
- Toppings: sliced fresh mango, kiwi, pineapple chunks, shredded coconut, chopped nuts, and a sprinkle of chia seeds

Instructions:

Blend frozen mango chunks, ripe banana, ground turmeric, orange juice, and Greek or coconut yogurt until homogeneous. Adjust consistency with more orange juice. Transfer mango-turmeric blend to a bowl and top with shredded coconut, nuts, pineapple, kiwi slices, fresh mango slices, almonds, and chia seeds. Enjoy the tropical flavors of your Mango Turmeric Sunshine Bowl, adjusting toppings and fruit to your taste. Enjoy the fun and healthy mix of mango and turmeric.

3. Acai Blueberry Bliss Bowl

Ingredients:

- 2 packs of frozen acai berry puree
- 1 cup frozen blueberries
- 1 ripe banana
- ½ cup almond milk (or any preferred milk)
- Toppings: granola, fresh blueberries, strawberries, sliced bananas, shredded coconut, chia seeds, and honey/agave syrup (optional)

Instructions:

To make the Acai Blueberry Bliss Bowl, blend frozen acai packs with frozen blueberries, ripe banana, and almond milk until smooth and creamy. Adjust the consistency by adding more milk if needed. Pour the blended acai mixture into a bowl and top with granola, fresh blueberries, sliced strawberries, banana slices, shredded coconut, and chia seeds. Optionally, drizzle honey or agave syrup for added sweetness. Enjoy immediately and adjust the toppings or proportions to your liking.

4. Spinach Pineapple Glow Bowl

Ingredients:

- 2 cups fresh spinach leaves
- 1 cup frozen pineapple chunks
- 1 ripe banana
- ½ cup plain or vanilla yogurt (regular or dairy-free)
- ½ cup coconut water or water
- Toppings: sliced fresh pineapple, kiwi, strawberries, shredded coconut, pumpkin seeds, and a drizzle of honey (optional)

Instructions:

To create a spinach pineapple glow bowl, blend fresh spinach leaves, frozen pineapple chunks, ripe banana, yogurt, and water or coconut water until homogeneous. Add more liquid if needed. Transfer the spinach-pineapple blend to a bowl and top with fresh pineapple, kiwi slices, halved strawberries, shredded coconut, pumpkin seeds, and honey. Enjoy the bright tastes and nourishing elements of your bowl immediately. Adjust the ratios or toppings to your preference, as these bowls are adaptable and can be customized to fit specific dietary requirements or personal tastes.

5. Kiwi Coconut Immunity Bowl

Ingredients:

- 2 ripe kiwis, peeled and sliced
- 1 cup coconut milk (canned or carton)
- ½ cup frozen pineapple chunks
- ½ cup frozen mango chunks
- ½ cup Greek yogurt or coconut yogurt
- Toppings: sliced kiwi, shredded coconut, granola, pumpkin seeds, and a drizzle of honey (optional)

Instructions:

This Kiwi Coconut Immunity Bowl is a delicious and nutritious way to support immunity. To make it, blend ripe kiwis, coconut milk, frozen pineapple, mango chunks, and Greek yogurt or coconut yogurt until smooth. Pour the mixture into a bowl, top with kiwi, shredded coconut, granola, pumpkin seeds, and honey for sweetness. Enjoy immediately and customize the toppings or ratios to suit your taste buds and nutritional needs.

C. Herbal Teas and Antioxidant Beverages

1. Chamomile Lavender Soothing Tea

Ingredients:

- 1 tablespoon dried chamomile flowers
- 1 teaspoon dried lavender buds
- 2 cups water
- Honey or a slice of lemon (optional, for sweetness or flavor)

Instructions:

This recipe involves preparing dried lavender buds and chamomile flowers in a teapot or heat proof container. Boil two cups of water to a boiling point, then cover the herbs and steep for five to seven minutes. Strain the tea into cups or a serving pot, adding honey or lemon for additional flavor. Enjoy this calming tea, perfect for winding down and relaxation. Chamomile and lavender are known for their relaxing qualities, making it a great option for quiet evenings or peace of mind. Adjust the amount of herbs to suit your taste.

2. Rooibos Hibiscus Antioxidant Infusion

Ingredients:

- 2 teaspoons Rooibos tea leaves
- 1 teaspoon dried hibiscus flowers
- 2 cups water

- Optional: honey or a squeeze of lemon for added sweetness or flavor

Instructions:

This is a recipe for a Rooibos Hibiscus Infusion, made by combining dried hibiscus flowers and Rooibos tea leaves in a heat proof container. Boil two cups of water and transfer the mixture to the teapot or container. Steep for five to seven minutes, allowing the flavors and antioxidants to seep into the water. Strain the infusion to remove the tea leaves and blossoms. Customize the infusion with lemon or honey for sweetness or flavor. Enjoy this antioxidant-rich infusion, which is known for its health benefits and delicious taste. Adjust the brewing time or ingredients to suit your personal taste.

3. Matcha Mint Green Elixir

Ingredients:

- 1 teaspoon matcha powder
- 1 cup hot water (not boiling, around 175°F or 80°C)
- 3-4 fresh mint leaves
- Honey or sweetener of choice (optional)

Instructions:

To make a Matcha Mint Green Elixir, combine matcha powder, hot water, mint leaves, and a small whisk or spoon. Use a bamboo whisk or small whisk to mix the ingredients until smooth. Add mint leaves and let them steep for 1-2 minutes. Strain the drink to remove mint leaves and add honey or a sweetener of your choice for a sweeter taste. Enjoy the refreshing and invigorating Matcha Mint Green Elixir, which combines earthy flavors of matcha with the refreshing essence of mint, making it perfect for a morning boost or midday pick-me-up. Adjust mint or sweetness levels according to your taste preferences.

4. Elderberry Rosehip Immune Booster

Ingredients:

- 1 cup dried elderberries
- 1/2 cup dried rosehips
- 4 cups water
- 1 cup honey (or adjust to taste)

Instructions:

In a medium saucepan, combine dried elderberries, rosehips, and water. Bring to a boil, then reduce heat and simmer for 30 to 45 minutes. Remove from heat and let cool to room temperature. Strain the liquid using cheesecloth or mesh, then add honey while it's still warm. Stir until all honey dissolves. Transfer the syrup to glass bottles or jars and refrigerate.

5. *Ginger Lemon Detox Elixir*

Ingredients:

- 1 inch piece of fresh ginger, peeled and sliced
- 1 lemon, juiced
- 4 cups water
- Optional: honey or maple syrup for sweetness

Instructions:

To prepare a Ginger Lemon Detox Elixir, peel and slice fresh ginger into thin pieces. Boil 4 cups of water in a pot, add the sliced ginger, reduce heat to low, and let it simmer for 10-15 minutes. Squeeze the lemon juice into the water, and add honey or maple syrup if desired. Strain the elixir to remove the ginger pieces. Enjoy this cleansing and zesty detox elixir, known for its cleansing properties and zesty taste. Enjoy the Ginger Lemon Detox Elixir for its cleansing properties and zesty taste.

CHAPTER 7: MEAL PLANS FOR LASTING YOUTH

7-Day Anti-Aging Meal Plan

Day 1:

Breakfast: Superfood Smoothie Bowl with Mixed Berries, Spinach, Chia Seeds, and Almond Milk.

Ingredients:

- 1 cup mixed berries (strawberries, blueberries, raspberries)
- 1 cup fresh spinach leaves
- 2 tablespoons chia seeds
- 1 cup almond milk (adjust quantity for desired consistency)
- Optional toppings: sliced fruits, nuts, seeds, granola

Instructions:

To create a nutritious superfood smoothie bowl, wash berries and spinach thoroughly. Blend mixed berries, spinach leaves, chia seeds, and almond milk until smooth in a blender. Adjust almond milk if needed. Pour into a bowl and top with additional berries, fruits, nuts, seeds, or granola for texture. Enjoy your nutritious and delicious bowl, adjusting ingredient quantities to suit your taste and dietary needs.

Lunch: Quinoa Salad with Avocado, Cherry Tomatoes, Cucumber, and a Lemon-Tahini Dressing.

Ingredients:

- 1 cup quinoa, rinsed
- 2 cups water or vegetable broth
- 1 avocado, diced
- 1 cup cherry tomatoes, halved
- 1 cucumber, diced
- 2 tablespoons chopped fresh parsley (optional)

For the Lemon-Tahini Dressing:

- 3 tablespoons tahini
- Juice of 1-2 lemons (adjust to taste)
- 2 tablespoons olive oil
- 1 garlic clove, minced

- Salt and pepper to taste
- Water (to adjust consistency)

Instructions:

Prepare quinoa according to the box's instructions and let it cool. Mix cooked quinoa, avocado, cherry tomatoes, cucumber, and parsley in a large bowl. Add tahini, lemon juice, olive oil, garlic, salt, and pepper. Gradually add water to achieve desired consistency. Cover the salad with the Lemon-Tahini Dressing and gently toss. Taste and adjust spices as needed. Serve cold or room temperature. Add other ingredients for texture and nutrition, such as almonds, feta cheese, or chickpeas. Enjoy the flavor and nutrition of this quinoa salad.

Dinner: Baked Salmon with Dill and Asparagus, served with a side of Roasted Sweet Potatoes.

Ingredients:

- 4 salmon filets
- 1 bunch of asparagus, trimmed
- 2 tablespoons olive oil
- Salt and pepper to taste
- 2 tablespoons chopped fresh dill
- Lemon wedges for serving

Roasted Sweet Potatoes

- 3-4 medium sweet potatoes, peeled and diced
- 2 tablespoons olive oil
- 1 teaspoon paprika
- Salt and pepper to taste
- Chopped fresh parsley for garnish (optional)

Instructions:

Preheat your oven to 400°F (200°C) and place salmon filets on a baking sheet. Arrange trimmed asparagus around the salmon, drizzle olive oil over them, season with salt and pepper, and sprinkle fresh dill. Bake for 12-15 minutes until cooked through and easily flakes. Remove from the oven and serve with lemon wedges.

 Preheat your oven to 425°F (220°C) and toss diced sweet potatoes with olive oil, paprika, salt, and pepper. Spread them on a baking sheet and roast for 25-30 minutes until tender and golden brown. Garnish with fresh parsley if desired. Serve the salmon and asparagus with the roasted sweet potatoes for a delicious and nutritious meal.

Day 2:

Breakfast: Protein-Packed Pancakes with Fresh Blueberries and a drizzle of Honey.

Ingredients:

- 1 cup oats (or oat flour)
- 1 ripe banana
- 2 eggs
- 1/2 cup Greek yogurt
- 1 teaspoon baking powder
- 1/2 teaspoon vanilla extract
- Pinch of salt
- Butter or oil for cooking

Toppings:

- Fresh blueberries
- Honey

Instructions:

To make high-protein pancakes, process oats in a food processor into flour and mix with ripe banana, Greek yogurt, eggs, baking powder, vanilla essence, and salt. Gradually stir the oat flour into the wet ingredients until smooth. If too thick, add milk. Heat a nonstick pan or griddle over medium heat and pour 1/4 cup of batter onto it. Fry until bubbles appear and cook until both sides are golden brown.

Garnish with fresh blueberries and drizzle with honey for a delightful garnish. Enjoy these pancakes for a delicious breakfast or brunch, topped with fresh blueberries and a hint of honey.

Lunch: Mediterranean Chickpea Salad with Kalamata Olives, Cherry Tomatoes, Feta Cheese, and a Balsamic Vinaigrette.

Mediterranean Chickpea Salad

Ingredients:

- 2 cans (15 oz each) chickpeas, drained and rinsed
- 1 cup cherry tomatoes, halved
- 1/2 cup Kalamata olives, pitted and sliced
- 1/2 cup crumbled feta cheese
- 1/4 cup chopped fresh parsley
- 1/4 cup chopped red onion (optional)

Balsamic Vinaigrette:

- 3 tablespoons balsamic vinegar
- 1/4 cup extra-virgin olive oil
- 1 teaspoon Dijon mustard
- 1 clove garlic, minced
- Salt and pepper to taste

Instructions:

This Mediterranean Chickpea Salad is a refreshing and flavorful dish that can be served as a side or a light, healthy meal on its own. It consists of chickpeas, cherry tomatoes, Kalamata olives, crumbled feta cheese, parsley, and red onion. The vinaigrette is made by whisking balsamic vinegar, extra-virgin olive oil, Dijon mustard, minced garlic, salt, and pepper. The salad is then tossed to coat all ingredients evenly. Adjusting seasoning if needed is recommended before serving.

Dinner: Grilled Lemon Herb Chicken with Quinoa and Steamed Broccoli.

Grilled Lemon Herb Chicken

Ingredients:

- 4 boneless, skinless chicken breasts
- 2 tablespoons olive oil
- Zest and juice of 1 lemon
- 2 cloves garlic, minced
- 1 teaspoon dried oregano
- 1 teaspoon dried thyme
- Salt and pepper to taste

Quinoa and Steamed Broccoli:

- 1 cup quinoa, rinsed
- 2 cups water or chicken broth
- 1 head of broccoli, cut into florets

Instructions:

Create a marinade by combining olive oil, lemon zest, lemon juice, garlic, oregano, thyme, salt, and pepper. Cover chicken breasts in the marinade and refrigerate for 30 minutes. Grill on medium-high for 6-8 minutes on each side, cooking time varying based on chicken thickness. Prepare quinoa according to package directions, adding flavor with water or chicken stock. Steam broccoli for 5-7 minutes until soft but crunchy. Serve the grilled lemon herb chicken with cooked quinoa and steamed broccoli for a nutrient-rich dinner. Enjoy!

Day 3:

Breakfast: Chia Pudding Power Bowl topped with Sliced Almonds and Mixed Berries.

Ingredients:

- 1/4 cup chia seeds

- 1 cup almond milk (or any preferred milk)
- 1 tablespoon maple syrup or honey (optional, for sweetness)
- 1/2 teaspoon vanilla extract
- Sliced almonds for topping
- Mixed berries (such as strawberries, blueberries, raspberries) for topping

Instructions:

To make a Chia Pudding Power Bowl, combine chia seeds, almond milk, vanilla essence, maple syrup, or honey in a jar or dish. Stir to fully blend. Cover and refrigerate for at least two hours or overnight to help the chia seeds absorb the liquid. Once set, transfer the pudding to a dish and top with chopped almonds and mixed berries for crunch and antioxidants. This filling and healthy breakfast or snack option contains omega-3 fatty acids from chia seeds, as well as the benefits of fresh berries and almonds.

Lunch: Spinach and White Bean Soup with a side of Whole Grain Bread.

Ingredients:

- 2 tablespoons olive oil
- 1 onion, chopped

- 3 cloves garlic, minced
- 4 cups vegetable or chicken broth
- 2 cans (15 oz each) white beans, drained and rinsed
- 4 cups fresh spinach, roughly chopped
- 1 teaspoon dried thyme
- Salt and pepper to taste
- Red pepper flakes (optional, for added heat)
- Freshly grated Parmesan cheese for serving (optional)

Instructions:

In a large pot, sauté onion and garlic in olive oil. Add vegetable or chicken broth and drained white beans, simmering for 10-15 minutes. Add thyme, salt, pepper, and red pepper flakes, and let the soup meld. Stir in fresh spinach and cook for 2-3 minutes until wilted. Taste and adjust seasoning if needed. Serve this Spinach and White Bean Soup hot with whole grain bread for a satisfying meal. Garnish with freshly grated Parmesan cheese for added flavor.

Dinner: Vegan Lentil and Vegetable Stir-Fry with Brown Rice.

Ingredients:

- 1 cup brown rice (uncooked)
- 1 ½ cups cooked lentils (you can use canned lentils or cook them beforehand)
- 2 tablespoons sesame oil or olive oil
- 3 cloves garlic, minced
- 1 onion, thinly sliced
- 2 cups mixed vegetables (such as bell peppers, broccoli, carrots, snap peas)
- ½ cup sliced mushrooms
- 3 tablespoons soy sauce or tamari
- 1 tablespoon rice vinegar
- 1 tablespoon maple syrup or agave syrup
- 1 teaspoon grated ginger
- Sesame seeds for garnish (optional)
- Chopped green onions for garnish (optional)

Instructions:

This recipe involves preparing brown rice, sautéing onion slices and garlic in sesame oil, then adding mushrooms and vegetables. Stir-fry for a few minutes until crisp and tender. In a separate bowl, combine rice vinegar, soy sauce, maple syrup, and ginger. Add cooked lentils and sauce to the vegetables, stir, and cook for two to three minutes. Top brown rice with the stir-fried lentils and vegetables, and garnish with chopped green onions and sesame seeds for added flavor. This healthy, high-protein vegan stir-fried dish is a delicious and nutritious choice for a healthy meal.

Day 4:

Breakfast: Greek Yogurt Parfait with Granola, Mixed Berries, and a drizzle of Honey.

Ingredients:

- 1 cup Greek yogurt (plain or flavored)
- 1/2 cup granola
- 1/2 cup mixed berries (such as strawberries, blueberries, raspberries)
- Honey for drizzling

Instructions:

This recipe involves layering Greek yogurt, granola, mixed berries, and honey in a glass or bowl. The yogurt is topped with granola, followed by mixed berries. The yogurt is then drizzled with honey for sweetness. The top is topped with mixed berries. The parfait can be customized with nuts, seeds, or cinnamon for extra flavor. This recipe is a healthy and satisfying breakfast or snack option.

Lunch: Caprese Stuffed Portobello Mushrooms served with a side of Mixed Greens.

Caprese Stuffed Portobello Mushrooms

Ingredients:

- 4 large Portobello mushrooms, stems removed
- 2 large tomatoes, sliced
- 1 ball fresh mozzarella cheese, sliced
- Fresh basil leaves
- Balsamic glaze (optional)
- Olive oil
- Salt and pepper to taste

Mixed Greens Side:

- Mixed salad greens
- Balsamic vinaigrette or preferred dressing

Instructions:

Preheat the oven to 375°F (190°C). Clean and remove stems from Portobello mushrooms, brush with olive oil, and sprinkle with salt and pepper. Place mushrooms on a baking sheet, gill side up. Layer with tomato, mozzarella, and basil leaves. Drizzle olive oil over each mushroom. Bake for 15-20 minutes until the cheese is melted and tender.

Optionally, drizzle with balsamic glaze for added flavor.

Mixed Greens Side:

Mix mixed salad greens with your preferred dressing and serve Caprese Stuffed Portobello Mushrooms alongside them for a satisfying meal. This dish pairs Portobello mushrooms, tomatoes, fresh mozzarella, and basil, creating a delightful and satisfying meal complemented by the freshness of mixed greens on the side.

Dinner: Teriyaki Glazed Mahi-Mahi with Quinoa and Stir-Fried Vegetables.

Teriyaki Glazed Mahi-Mahi

 Ingredients:

- 4 Mahi-Mahi filets
- 1/4 cup teriyaki sauce
- 2 tablespoons soy sauce
- 2 tablespoons honey
- 2 cloves garlic, minced
- 1 tablespoon sesame oil (for cooking)
- Sesame seeds for garnish (optional)
- Chopped green onions for garnish (optional)

Quinoa:

- 1 cup quinoa, rinsed
- 2 cups water or vegetable broth
- Salt to taste

Stir-Fried Vegetables:

- Assorted vegetables (such as bell peppers, broccoli, carrots, snap peas)
- 1 tablespoon olive oil
- 2 cloves garlic, minced
- 2 tablespoons soy sauce
- Salt and pepper to taste

Instructions:

To prepare a Teriyaki Glazed Mahi-Mahi, start by preheating your oven to 375°F or 190°C. In a bowl, mix teriyaki sauce, soy sauce, honey, and garlic. Transfer the Mahi-Mahi filets to a shallow dish and cover with the marinade. Refrigerate for 20-30 minutes. Cook the quinoa according to the package, adding more flavor with water or vegetable broth. Meanwhile, prepare the vegetables for stir-frying in olive oil and seasoning with pepper, salt, and soy sauce. Preheat the sesame oil in an oven-safe skillet and sear the marinated Mahi-Mahi filets for 2-3 minutes on each side. Place the pan in the oven and bake for another 5-7 minutes until the fish is well cooked and flakeable. Serve the stir-fried veggies and Teriyaki Glazed Mahi over the quinoa, and garnish with chopped green onions and sesame seeds if desired.

Day 5:

Breakfast: Oat and Goji Berry Breakfast Bowl with Almond Butter and Banana Slices.

Ingredients:

- ½ cup rolled oats
- 1 cup almond milk (or any preferred milk)
- 2 tablespoons goji berries
- 1 tablespoon almond butter
- 1 banana, sliced
- Optional: honey or maple syrup for sweetness

Instructions:

This recipe involves preparing rolled oats and almond milk in a pot, stirring regularly over medium heat until the mixture reaches desired consistency. While the oatmeal is still warm, stir in goji berries to soften them. Spoon the cooked oatmeal and goji berries onto a serving dish, drizzle with almond butter, and top with banana slices. If desired, drizzle more honey or maple syrup for extra sweetness. This nutritious breakfast bowl is packed with fiber, antioxidants from goji berries, and good fats from almond butter. Other toppings like nuts, seeds, or cinnamon can be added for taste. Adjust the sweetness to suit your preference.

Lunch: Watermelon and Feta Salad with Mint and a Balsamic Glaze.

Ingredients:

- Cubed watermelon
- Feta cheese, crumbled or cubed
- Fresh mint leaves, chopped
- Balsamic glaze or reduction

Instructions:

This recipe involves preparing a watermelon and feta salad. Cut the watermelon into cubes and crumble the cheese. Arrange the cubed watermelon and feta in a serving bowl or platter. Add mint leaves and drizzle with balsamic glaze for a sweet tanginess. Finish with a touch of freshly cracked black pepper for an extra flavor dimension. This light, vibrant salad is perfect for summer, with a mix of sweet, savory, and refreshing flavors. Adjust the ingredients according to your preference and enjoy this summer salad.

Dinner: Turmeric and Ginger Lentil Stew with a side of Cauliflower Rice.

Ingredients:

- 1 cup dried lentils (rinsed)
- 1 tablespoon olive oil or coconut oil
- 1 onion, diced
- 2 cloves garlic, minced
- 1-inch piece of ginger, grated
- 1 teaspoon ground turmeric
- ½ teaspoon ground cumin
- 4 cups vegetable broth or water
- Salt and pepper to taste
- Fresh cilantro for garnish (optional)
- 1 head cauliflower, grated or processed into rice-like texture
- Olive oil
- Salt and pepper to taste

Instructions:

This recipe involves preparing dry lentils by rinsing them under running water. In a large saucepan, sauté aromatics by heating olive oil over medium heat. Add onion slices and grated ginger and minced garlic, and simmer for a minute or so. Add ground cumin and turmeric, stir, and stir the washed lentils into the mixture. Fill the saucepan with water or vegetable broth, bring to a boil, then simmer for 20-25 minutes.

Next, assemble cauliflower rice by grating or pulsing it until it resembles rice. In a pan over medium heat, sprinkle olive oil and add the cauliflower rice. Simmer for 5-7 minutes, stirring occasionally. Season with salt and pepper to taste.

Serve the Turmeric and Ginger Lentil Stew in bowls, top with fresh cilantro, and serve with cauliflower rice for a hearty and tasty supper. Adjust the spice or add other veggies to suit your taste. This meal is full of fiber, protein, and bright flavors from the ginger and turmeric.

Day 6:

Breakfast: Acai Berry Bliss Bowl topped with Coconut Flakes and Granola.

Ingredients:

- 2 packs frozen acai berry puree
- 1 banana, frozen (optional for creaminess)
- ½ cup frozen mixed berries
- ½ cup almond milk (or any preferred milk)
- Toppings: coconut flakes, granola, fresh berries, sliced banana, chia seeds (optional)

Instructions:

This recipe for an Acai Berry Bliss Bowl with Granola and Coconut Flakes involves blending frozen acai packets with almond milk, mixed berries, and frozen banana. The mixture is then puréed until creamy and smooth, with the possibility of adding more almond milk if needed. The pureed acai mixture is then topped with granola and coconut flakes, sliced banana, fresh berries, and chia seeds for texture. This high-nutrient breakfast or snack is rich in fiber, antioxidants, and good fats. To customize the toppings, nuts, seeds, or honey can be added for sweetness. Enjoy the bright tastes and filling deliciousness of this delicious bowl.

Lunch: Chickpea and Spinach Stuffed Bell Peppers.

Ingredients:

- 4 large bell peppers, tops removed and seeds removed
- 1 can (15 oz) chickpeas, drained and rinsed
- 2 cups fresh spinach, chopped
- 1 small onion, finely chopped
- 2 cloves garlic, minced
- 1 teaspoon ground cumin
- 1 teaspoon paprika
- Salt and pepper to taste
- 1 cup cooked quinoa or rice
- 1/2 cup shredded cheese (optional, for topping)
- Fresh parsley or cilantro for garnish (optional)

Instructions:

Preheat the oven to 375°F or 190°C. Heat olive oil in a skillet over medium heat. Add onion and garlic, sauté, then add chickpeas and chopped spinach. Season with salt, pepper, paprika, and ground cumin. Add cooked rice or quinoa and stuff the mixture into each bell pepper. Transfer the filled peppers to a baking tray and cover with foil. Bake for 25-30 minutes or until soft. Melt cheese may be added in the last five minutes of baking. Garnish with fresh cilantro or parsley before serving. These stuffed bell peppers with chickpeas and spinach are a filling and healthy supper.

Dinner: Quinoa and Roasted Vegetable Salad with Lemon-Herb Dressing.

Ingredients:

For the Salad:

- 1 cup quinoa, rinsed
- Assorted vegetables (such as bell peppers, zucchini, cherry tomatoes, red onion)
- 2 tablespoons olive oil
- Salt and pepper to taste
- Fresh herbs (such as thyme, rosemary, or parsley), chopped for garnish

For the Lemon-Herb Dressing:

- 1/4 cup olive oil
- Juice of 1-2 lemons (depending on desired tartness)
- 2 cloves garlic, minced
- 1 teaspoon Dijon mustard
- 1 tablespoon honey or maple syrup (optional for sweetness)
- 1 teaspoon dried herbs (such as oregano, basil, or thyme)
- Salt and pepper to taste

Instructions:

This recipe involves roasting vegetables at 400°F or 200°C, chopping them into small pieces, arranging them on a baking sheet, adding salt and pepper, and drizzling with olive oil. Roast the vegetables for 20-25 minutes until they are soft and caramelized. Prepare the quinoa according to the package directions, fluff it up, and let it cool to room temperature. In a small bowl, whisk together olive oil, lemon juice, dried herbs, Dijon mustard, minced garlic, honey or maple syrup, salt, and pepper. Combine the roasted veggies and cooked quinoa in a large bowl, drizzle with the lemon-herb dressing, toss lightly, and sprinkle with freshly cut herbs before serving. This colorful salad is perfect for a main meal or a side dish.

Day 7:

Breakfast: Green Superfood Smoothie Bowl with Kale, Pineapple, and Chia Seeds.

Ingredients:

- 1 cup kale leaves, stems removed and chopped
- 1 cup frozen pineapple chunks
- 1 ripe banana, frozen or fresh
- 1/2 cup almond milk (or any preferred milk)

- 1 tablespoon chia seeds
- Toppings: Sliced fresh fruits, nuts, seeds, granola, coconut flakes (optional)

Instructions:

Blend frozen pineapple chunks, ripe banana, kale leaves, almond milk, and chia seeds until creamy and smooth. Add extra almond milk if needed. Transfer the smoothie to a bowl and top with sliced fresh fruits. For texture, add almonds, seeds, granola, or coconut flakes. Enjoy this nutrient-rich Green Superfood Smoothie Bowl for a hydrating breakfast or snack.

Lunch: Asian-Inspired Cucumber and Sesame Salad with Grilled Tofu.

Ingredients:

- 1 block of firm tofu, pressed and sliced
- 2 tablespoons soy sauce or tamari
- 1 tablespoon sesame oil
- 1 tablespoon rice vinegar
- 1 teaspoon grated ginger
- 1 clove garlic, minced
- Salt and pepper to taste
- Cooking oil for grilling
- 2 cucumbers, thinly sliced

- 2 tablespoons rice vinegar
- 1 tablespoon soy sauce or tamari
- 1 teaspoon sesame oil
- 1 teaspoon honey or maple syrup (optional for sweetness)
- 1 tablespoon sesame seeds
- Sliced green onions or cilantro for garnish (optional)

Instructions:

To prepare a delicious Asian-inspired cucumber and sesame salad, marinate the tofu in rice vinegar, sesame oil, grated ginger, garlic, soy sauce or tamari, salt, and pepper for at least half an hour. Heat a grill pan or skillet over medium-high heat and cook the marinated tofu for 3-4 minutes on each side. Meanwhile, prepare thinly sliced cucumbers and prepare a dressing made from rice vinegar, sesame oil, soy sauce or tamari, honey or maple syrup. Cover the cucumber slices with the dressing, toss them thoroughly, scatter sesame seeds, and garnish with cilantro or green onions. Serve the salad with the grilled tofu for a savory, light, and satisfying supper. You can add red pepper flakes or change the flavors to give it a kick. Enjoy this tasty and nutritious meal.

Dinner: Baked Chicken Breast with Sweet Potato Mash and Steamed Green Beans.

Ingredients:

Baked Chicken Breast

- 2 boneless, skinless chicken breasts
- Olive oil
- Salt, pepper, and preferred seasoning (such as paprika, garlic powder, or herbs)

Mashed Sweet Potato

- 2 medium-sized sweet potatoes, peeled and cubed
- Butter or olive oil
- Salt and pepper to taste

Steamed Green Beans:
- Fresh green beans, trimmed
- Salt

Instructions:

Preheat the oven to 400°F or 200°C. Season chicken breasts with salt, pepper, and your preferred spice blend. Place the seasoned chicken in a baking dish or on a baking sheet covered with parchment paper.

Bake for 20-25 minutes until the internal temperature reaches 165°F (74°C).

Cook diced potatoes in boiling water for 15-20 minutes until soft. Mash the potatoes with a fork or potato masher and combine butter or olive oil with salt and pepper for seasoning.
Steam green beans in a steamer basket over boiling water until crisp-tender, around 4-5 minutes.

Serve the Baked Chicken Breast on a plate with steamed green beans and sweet potato mash. This nutrient-dense, well-balanced meal is full of fiber and protein. Add herbs or garlic for flavor and olive oil or lemon zest for a finishing touch. Enjoy your filling and healthy dinner!

CHAPTER 8: TIPS AND TRICKS FOR A FOREVER YOUNG LIFESTYLE

Choosing nutrient-dense foods high in antioxidants, vitamins, minerals, and other components that promote general health and combat oxidative stress is an intelligent grocery shopping strategy for anti-aging. Here's how to buy wisely for groceries to prevent aging:

1. Brightly colored fruits and vegetables: Select a range of vibrant fruits and vegetables, such as bell peppers, carrots, spinach, kale, and berries. They have a lot of antioxidants, which fight against free radicals.

2. Berries: Select blueberries, strawberries, raspberries, and blackberries from the list of berries. They contain anti-inflammatory qualities and are loaded with antioxidants.

3. Fatty Fish: Incorporate fish that are high in fat, such as sardines, mackerel, and salmon. They include a lot of omega-3 fatty acids, which promote healthy skin and lower inflammation.

4. Nuts and Seeds: Choose chia seeds, flaxseeds, walnuts, and almonds. They include fiber, vital minerals, and good fats.

5. Whole Grains: Opt for whole grains such as oats, brown rice, and quinoa. They include dietary fiber, vitamins, and minerals that are vital for healthy skin and general wellbeing.

6. Lean Proteins: Choose lean protein sources including lentils, beans, tofu, and chicken. Collagen synthesis and tissue healing depend on protein.

7. Green Tea: Add this tea, which is high in antioxidants. It could aid in enhancing skin elasticity and shielding the skin from UV rays.

8. Olive Oil: When cooking, use extra virgin olive oil. It has antioxidants and monounsaturated fats that support heart health and may be good for the skin.

9. Vibrant Herbs and Spices: Include on your shopping list herbs like cinnamon, ginger, and turmeric. These spices contain antioxidant and anti-inflammatory qualities.

10. Low-Fat Dairy or Dairy Alternatives: Select dairy products that are low in fat and/or calcium and vitamin D for healthy bones.

11. Hydration Sources: To remain hydrated, which is essential for keeping good skin, buy plenty of water, herbal teas, and coconut water.

12. Dark Chocolate: On rare occasions, treat yourself to dark chocolate that has at least 70% cacao. Flavonoids found in it may have anti-aging properties.

13. Vibrant Legumes: Incorporate a range of legumes, including lentils, black beans, and chickpeas. They provide a variety of minerals, fiber, and protein.

14. Greek Yogurt: Choose Greek yogurt to enhance digestive health and as a great source of protein and probiotics.

15. Avocado: Include avocados in your shopping list for their beneficial fats and vitamins that support the health of your skin.

ADVICE

- Give fresh, whole foods precedence over packaged and processed meals.
- Check food labels for added sugars and unhealthy fats.
- To get the freshest and healthiest products possible, choose seasonal and locally produced goods.

Recall that the secret to maximizing the advantages of anti-aging is a healthy lifestyle coupled with a diverse and balanced diet. Seek guidance from a qualified dietician or healthcare provider for individualized recommendations based on your unique medical requirements.

CONCLUSION

Congratulations for finishing "The Quick and Easy Forever Strong Diet Cookbook!" You have set out to completely change the way you feel about food, making it a source of vigor and power while yet keeping it approachable and easy to use. When you wrap up this culinary journey, take a moment to consider the useful resources and engaging strategies that make this cookbook special and transformative.

Our goal in writing this book has been to create an immersive learning experience rather than merely recipes. Each component was meant to actively include you in your culinary decisions, in addition to just instructing you. Our goal is to make cooking more comfortable for you, from the vibrant pictures that go with the recipes to the useful advice on where to get ingredients and how to prepare meals.

There are no quick cures or radical adjustments involved in the Forever Strong Diet. It's a way of life based on strong principles that gives you the ability to choose your meals with knowledge. The significance of variety, balance, and nutrient content in every meal has been emphasized. You're setting the foundation for long-term health and wellbeing by implementing the ideas presented in this cookbook.

Although nutrition may be a complicated topic, we've made an effort to make it understandable and relevant to everybody. The Quick and Easy Forever Strong Diet Cookbook is for everyone who wants to adopt a healthier lifestyle without compromising taste or ease of use—not only seasoned cooks or nutrition aficionados. We have reduced the complexity of these ideas so that everyone can understand and use them.

Remember that this is not a farewell, but rather the start of a lifetime path toward health and wellbeing when you say goodbye to this cookbook. Take this book as a starting point and play around with the recipes, modifying them to your own preferences and adding your gained understanding to your everyday routine. Please feel free to share your insights, learnings, and modifications with the lively community of foodies and other readers.

This is only the beginning of your culinary adventure; there is always more to discover in terms of tastes, textures, and nutrition. Accept the many opportunities that lie ahead. Use this cookbook as a guide and source of inspiration to create delicious and nourishing meals that will nourish your body, mind, and spirit and leave you feeling strong for all time.

I am grateful that you shared in this life-changing event. Cheers to many more years of culinary exploration, good health, and pleasure!